Sheila D. Miller, DSW
Editor

C000133267

Disability
and the Black Community

Disability and the Black Community has been co-published simultaneously as *Journal of Health & Social Policy*, Volume 16, Numbers 1/2 2002.

*Pre-publication
REVIEWS,
COMMENTARIES,
EVALUATIONS . . .*

The Haworth Press, Inc.

Disability
and the Black Community

Disability and the Black Community has been co-published simultaneously as *Journal of Health & Social Policy*, Volume 16, Numbers 1/2 2002.

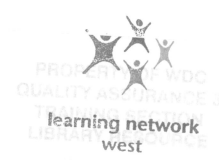

learning network
west

The *Journal of Health & Social Policy* Monographic "Separates"

Below is a list of " separates," which in serials librarianship means a special issue simultaneously published as a special journal issue or double-issue *and* as a "separate" hardbound monograph. (This is a format which we also call a "DocuSerial.")

"Separates" are published because specialized libraries or professionals may wish to purchase a specific thematic issue by itself in a format which can be separately cataloged and shelved, as opposed to purchasing the journal on an on-going basis. Faculty members may also more easily consider a "separate" for classroom adoption.

"Separates" are carefully classified separately with the major book jobbers so that the journal tie-in can be noted on new book order slips to avoid duplicate purchasing.

You may wish to visit Haworth's Website at . . .

http://www.HaworthPress.com

. . . to search our online catalog for complete tables of contents of these separates and related publications.

You may also call 1-800-HAWORTH (outside US/Canada: 607-722-5857), or Fax 1-800-895-0582 (outside US/Canada: 607-771-0012), or e-mail at:

docdelivery@haworthpress.com

Disability and the Black Community, *edited by Sheila D. Miller, DSW (Vol. 16, No. 1/2).* *"CONTAINS INSIGHTFUL DISCUSSIONS AND INNOVATIVE RECOMMENDATIONS and strategies. Dr. Miller has focused the collaborative efforts of twenty-two practitioners on the identification and advocacy of innovative methods to address the needs of the minority community for health care services and disability assurance." (Rheba G. Gwaltney, MA (Urban Education), Government Employee)*

Evaluation Research in Child Welfare: Improving Outcomes Through University-Public Agency Partnerships, edited by Katharine Briar-Lawson, PhD, and Joan Levy Zlotnik, PhD (Vol. 15, No. 3/4, 2002). *"TIMELY AND IMPORTANT, particularly in its emphasis on IV-E funded partnerships. NOT JUST FOR RESEARCHERS AND EVALUATORS. . . . Even readers who do not believe they are involved in evaluation will come to appreciate the essential relationship between evaluation and program design and implementation. Answering the questions 'How can we know whether our programs are effective?' and 'how can we improve effectiveness?' requires ongoing collaborative conversations among the full range of partnership participants. This book provides a good base from which to launch such conversations." (Lois Wright, MSSW, EdD, Assistant Dean, College of Social Work; Director, The Center for Child and Family Studies, University of South Carolina-Columbia)*

African-American Adolescents in the Urban Community: Social Services Policy and Practice Interventions, edited by Judith L. Rozie-Battle, MSW, JD (Vol. 15, No. 2, 2002). *"A comprehensive view of the challenges and opportunities that African-American youth face in today's changing society. . . . Shows that today's African-American youth face challenges that previous generations did not encounter. A must read." (Michael Bonds, PhD, Assistant Professor, Department of Educational Policy and Community Studies, University of Wisconsin-Milwaukee)*

Health and the American Indian, edited by Priscilla A. Day, MSW, and Hilary N. Weaver, DSW (Vol. 10, No. 4, 1999). *Discusses the health and mental health of Native American Indians from several aspects.*

Reason and Rationality in Health and Human Services Delivery, edited by John T. Pardeck, PhD, ACSW, Charles F. Longino, Jr., PhD, and John W. Murphy, PhD (Vol. 9, No. 4, 1998). *"A variety of perspectives that successfully challenge the pillars of modern medicine . . . . This book should be required of all health care professionals, especially those training to become physicians." (Roland Meinert, PhD, President, Missouri Association for Social Welfare, Jefferson City, Missouri)*

Selected Practical Problems in Health and Social Research, edited by Thomas E. Dinero, PhD (Vol. 8, No. 1, 1996). *"Explores some of the theoretical ideas underlying classical and modern* measurement theory. These ideas form a set of guidelines for researchers, health professionals, and students in the social, psychological, or health sciences who are planning and evaluating a measurement activity." (Inquiry)

Psychosocial Aspects of Sickle Cell Disease: Past, Present, and Future Directions of Research, edited by Kermit B. Nash, PhD (Vol. 5, No. 3/4, 1994). *"An excellent contribution to a neglected area of study and practice. . . . Offer[s] tools and techniques that one can easily incorporate into practice. Novice readers as well as seasoned practitioners will find the practicality of the book extremely helpful." (Social Work in Health Care)*

Health Care for the Poor and Uninsured: Strategies That Work, edited by Nellie P. Tate, PhD, and Kevin T. Kavanagh, MD, MS (Vol. 3, No. 4, 1992). *"Chapters are short and to the point with clearly defined goals, methods, techniques, and impacts and include easy-to-comprehend charts and statistics. This book will prove useful in understanding activities that may soon be an integral part of the American health care system." (Journal of Community Health)*

Published by

The Haworth Press, 10 Alice Street, Binghamton, NY 13904-1580

Disability and the Black Community has been co-published simultaneously as *Journal of Health & Social Policy*, Volume 16, Numbers 1/2 2002.

The development, preparation, and publication of this work has been undertaken with great care. However, the publisher, employees, editors, and agents of The Haworth Press and all imprints of The Haworth Press, Inc., including The Haworth Medical Press® and Pharmaceutical Products Press®, are not responsible for any errors contained herein or for consequences that may ensue from use of materials or information contained in this work. Opinions expressed by the author(s) are not necessarily those of The Haworth Press, Inc. With regard to case studies, identities and circumstances of individuals discussed herein have been changed to protect confidentiality. Any resemblance to actual persons, living or dead, is entirely coincidental.

Cover design by Jennifer M. Gaska

Library of Congress Cataloging-in-Publication Data

Disability and the black community / Sheila D. Miller, editor.
    p. ; cm.
    "Co-publisher simultaneously as Journal of health & social policy, volume 16, numbers 1/2."
    Includes bibliographical references and index.
    ISBN 0-7890-2076-9 (hard : paper)–ISBN 0-7890-2077-7 (pbk. : alk. paper)
    1. African Americans–Health and hygiene. 2. African Americans–Medical care. 3. Minority people with disabilities–Medical care–United States.
    [DNLM: 1. Disabled Persons–United States. 2. Health Policy–United States. 3. Blacks– United States. WA 540 AA1 D611 2002] I. Miller, Sheila D. II. Journal of health & social policy, volume 16, numbers 1/2.

RA448.5.N4D55 2002
362.1'089'96073–dc21

                                      2002155541

Disability
and the Black Community

Sheila D. Miller, DSW
Editor

Disability and the Black Community has been co-published simultaneously as *Journal of Health & Social Policy*, Volume 16, Numbers 1/2 2002.

The Haworth Press, Inc.
New York • London • Oxford

Indexing, Abstracting & Website/Internet Coverage

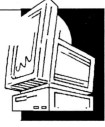

This section provides you with a list of major indexing & abstracting services. That is to say, each service began covering this periodical during the year noted in the right column. Most Websites which are listed below have indicated that they will either post, disseminate, compile, archive, cite or alert their own Website users with research-based content from this work. (This list is as current as the copyright date of this publication.)

Abstracting, Website/Indexing Coverage . . . . Year When Coverage Began

- *Abstracts in Anthropology* 1991

- *Abstracts in Social Gerontology: Current Literature on Aging.* 2000

- *Academic Abstracts/CD-ROM* 1994

- *AgeLine Database* 2000

- *c/o CAB International Access/CAB ACCESS <www.cabi.org>* 2002

- *Cambridge Scientific Abstracts (Health & Safety Science Abstracts/Risk Abstracts) <www.csa.com>* 1990

- *CNPIEC Reference Guide: Chinese National Directory of Foreign Periodicals* 1995

- *EMBASE/Excerpta Medica Secondary Publishing Division <URL: http://www.elsevier.nl>* 1992

- *Family & Society Studies Worldwide <www.nisc.com>* 1996

(continued)

(continued)

*Special Bibliographic Notes related to special journal issues
(separates) and indexing/abstracting:*

- indexing/abstracting services in this list will also cover material in any "separate" that is co-published simultaneously with Haworth's special thematic journal issue or DocuSerial. Indexing/abstracting usually covers material at the article/chapter level.
- monographic co-editions are intended for either non-subscribers or libraries which intend to purchase a second copy for their circulating collections.
- monographic co-editions are reported to all jobbers/wholesalers/approval plans. The source journal is listed as the "series" to assist the prevention of duplicate purchasing in the same manner utilized for books-in-series.
- to facilitate user/access services all indexing/abstracting services are encouraged to utilize the co-indexing entry note indicated at the bottom of the first page of each article/chapter/contribution.
- this is intended to assist a library user of any reference tool (whether print, electronic, online, or CD-ROM) to locate the monographic version if the library has purchased this version but not a subscription to the source journal.

Disability
and the Black Community

CONTENTS

ABOUT THE EDITOR

Sheila D. Miller, DSW, is a Professor in the Ethelyn R. Strong School of Social Work at Norfolk State University. She has published in the area of acceptance and adjustment to disability and has written in the area of significance of family support in the disabled African American community. She has provided regional and national presentations in the areas of illness, disability, rehabilitation, and in health issues confronting African American women. She has participated as a board member for the Council on Social Work Education, Commission on Disability and Persons with Disabilities, Society for the Aid of Sickle Cell Anemia, Friends of Norfolk Juvenile Court, Victims Against Crime, Inc. and, an Editorial Board member for the *Journal of Health & Social Policy*. She provided a review for the forthcoming publication, *Journal of Social Work in Disability & Rehabilitation* and reviewed a breast cancer manuscript for the Center for Research on Minority Health. Sheila Miller has provided consultations and chaired research in the areas of death and dying, grief and loss, criminal justice, substance abuse, domestic violence, sickle cell, hemodialysis, and welfare reform. The Judicial Council of Virginia certifies her in General District Court Mediation; and Juvenile and Domestic Relations District Court Mediation. Over the years, she has been a member of many social work, education and health organizations. She received awards in *Who's Who Among American Teachers*, in 1996 and 2000.

Preface

I am grateful to the Editors who gave me this opportunity to assemble this wonderful group of authors and address issues of disability in the Black community. I am honored to have the support of the researchers and professionals who have contributed to this book. This team represents a number of disciplines and regions. Their concern for the successful adjustment to disability of Black people is apparent. The collective years of practice, education and research are reflected in the articles and I appreciate the authors' commitment and dedication to the project.

This special volume is devoted to the Black disabled and their families. Our aim is to motivate, influence, and empower communities. Hopefully our efforts will assist in improving the environment and services of people facing disability. Understanding the complex nature and diversity of the Black disabled experience, this group of authors provides information that is useful for advocates trying to impact and educate larger systems.

Black communities have wonderful people on the front lines trying to aid the disabled and their families. The mission of helping the Black disabled and their families maintain dignity and self-worth is important and hard work. Social and political issues compound the ordeals confronting the Black disabled, and their advocates are determined to make recommendations and strategies available.

This volume will address a few of the many health issues and disabling situations confronting our community. It will require many more volumes of research to address all of the disabling situations confronting the Black community and we hope that others will join us in research efforts. We are aware that many disabled people have complicated health problems and that their disability status may be a result of other primary and secondary diagnoses. While it is recognized that some of the illnesses and disabilities may have an onset at very early ages, there are many others that become issues as a consequence of life situations, environmental, life styles, and stressors.

These wonderful selections attempt to assist racial and ethnic groups working with disabled Black people by providing research, models and paradigms. It is a way of helping others to effectively provide knowledge and improve interventions. Working towards acceptance and respect for the Black disabled community is the challenge and these authors have responded.

Sheila D. Miller, DSW

[Haworth co-indexing entry note]: "Preface." Miller. Sheila D. Co-published simultaneously in *Journal of Health & Social Policy* (The Haworth Press, Inc.) Vol. 16, No. 1/2, 2002, p. xix; and: *Disability and the Black Community* (ed: Sheila D. Miller) The Haworth Press, Inc., 2002, p. xv. Single or multiple copies of this article are available for a fee from The Haworth Document Delivery Service [1-800-HAWORTH, 9:00 a.m. - 5:00 p.m. (EST). E-mail address: docdelivery@haworthpress.com].

Acknowledgments

This volume is the result of many dedicated people who share a commitment to persons with disabilities and their families. I am very grateful for their hard work and enthusiasm for helping me to provide an exciting and provocative volume on disability issues in the black community. I am honored to have the experience of working with this wonderful team of professionals and indebted to them for providing their excellent work. I extend sincere appreciation to Marvin D. Feit and Stanley F. Battle, editors of the *Journal of Health & Social Policy* for this wonderful opportunity to address disability issues experienced in the black community.

I am thankful for having known Dr. Ethelyn R. Strong who mentored my early years of health and disability practice. Gratitude is extended to Dr. Joan Conway, and Mrs. Catherine Nelson, who nurture my interest in disability issues in minority communities and continue to encourage my commitment to physical and mental health. Thanks are, also, extended to the many agencies, data archives, and resource systems that provided data for the wonderful research provided in these articles.

I am very appreciative to my family and friends who provide support and encouragement. I am indebted to my sister, Mrs. Wanda Miller Nutall, who taught me the importance of understanding and respecting the disabled. Although it has been eleven years since she has transitioned, I am still moved by her courage and strength.

I would be remiss if I did not thank my friends, Elijah Mickel and Ruby Gourdine for their many years of support for all of my projects. Finally, the completion of this project was timely thanks to my favorite mail lady, Ms. Thelma Boards, who delivered the manuscripts with humor and best wishes from the post office.

Sheila D. Miller, DSW

Introduction

The contributors have provided articles for this volume demonstrating their knowledge and experience of disability and disabling situations in the Black community. It is hoped that this information will help the professional community to assist the communities where our disabled families and friends live. The disability situation is a part of many lives and the articles address a few of the many disability situations found in the community, and in the workplace. The goal for this volume is to increase the understanding and awareness of people working with the disabled. It is thought that this book will mobilize advocates, provide alternatives for successful intervention and planning, and encourage research in disability and rehabilitation.

It is important to note that the articles are in accordance with the broadening of the definition of disability as supported by the American Disabilities Act. The authors' discussions of the disability topics and issues provide a realistic understanding of the disabled experience and include recommendations for service providers. It is essential to acknowledge the hardships, the strengths and the determination of the Black disabled and their families to survive. This is reflected in the practice wisdoms and current research findings as they share their positions and provide alternatives.

This special volume addresses physical, mental, and learning disabilities that are experienced across, age, gender and ethnic groups in the Black race. The themes include selected physical disabilities, disabled children learning and program concerns, welfare reform, disabled public housing issues, domestic violence and disability curriculum content. There is much to be done, explored and researched in these areas and it is anticipated that many more scholars and researchers will become more involved in disability and rehabilitation initiatives.

[Haworth co-indexing entry note]: "Introduction." Miller, Sheila D. Co-published simultaneously in *Journal of Health & Social Policy* (The Haworth Press, Inc.) Vol. 16, No. 1/2, 2002, pp. 1-3; and: *Disability and the Black Community* (ed: Sheila D. Miller) The Haworth Press, Inc., 2002, pp. 1-3. Single or multiple copies of this article are available for a fee from The Haworth Document Delivery Service [1-800-HAWORTH, 9:00 a.m. - 5:00 p.m. (EST). E-mail address: docdelivery@haworthpress.com].

http://www.haworthpress.com/store/product.asp?sku=J045
10.1300/J045v16n01_01

The physical disability topics reflect the authors' most recent advance study and research interest. The diagnosis is of such magnitude that physical functioning is impaired. Symptoms may be inconsistent or constant which further impact the disabled person's life. The welfare reform topics are on the cutting edge of discussions and debates. In light of political and economic considerations, this topic affects all consumers as we strive to find genuine ways to provide quality life opportunities to disability patients. The influence that welfare and public housing have on the community is overwhelming many of the disabled persons and the people trying to help. The difficulty of the expectation of patient, family and advocate is overwhelming. The passion and commitment to challenge and help are evident in this contribution.

Themes on learning disabilities, academic achievements and mental health issues of children are presented. The themes incorporated the reality of learning disability and its multiple effects on children and families. Family and community debate as to the extent the academic environment is affected. The authors present exciting and innovative ideas that are helpful in understanding and helping in the complicated educational and learning dilemma of securing academic achievement.

Another unique and provocative article addresses health disparities and access to care. The authors present fascinating data, results and recommendations for health care and maintenance organizations. Access to care is a reoccurring theme and the dilemma is handled expertly in this wonderful article. The use of geographical data to identify disparities is exciting and expertly reinforces the authors' intent to galvanize health organizations to move to action.

There is a connection of protective factors and domestic violence that is important in understanding the domestic violence we observe in families. The domestic violence concerns are identified across systems and many times contribute to physical, mental and learning disability issues and crises. Domestic violence has far reaching implications and we have only begun to touch on the effects it has in our communities. This article helps us to broaden our thinking and develop new ideas and approaches for helping.

Finally, three articles present models recommended for aiding the disabled dilemma. They are practice, program and curriculum models resulting from extensive practice and research experience. The practice paradigm presented with an African-centered perspective is excellent as an alternative for work with Black patients and families. It addresses the significance of helping and healing techniques that support and reinforce the strengths already found in the Black community. The program model presented is of great importance to people working with disabled children. The recommendations for goals, services offered, procedures for successful program operation and services are carefully explained. It offers and appears to enhance the opportunities for the success of the disabled children. The model allows for flexibility for similar agencies to modify and to accommodate their unique program objectives. With extensive discussion on diversity in social work education, a research study is presented that suggests the inclusion of disability content in social work curriculum without threatening existing curriculum and program goals. Recognizing that disability issues overlap in all problem and practice areas, the study is timely and relevant. The additional knowledge will prepare the new professional for realistic practice in a changing world.

The contributing authors have presented their unique perspective of complex and diverse disability concerns. The quest for continuing to increase the success of adjustment for the disabled and their families is encouraged. Readers will find this volume stimulating and useful. The perseverance of these wonderful authors is inspirational and refreshing. I am grateful to them and extend thanks for their many hours of work providing me with their manuscripts. I applaud their years of hard work in assisting with disability issues in the Black community.

Sheila D. Miller, DSW

A Study to Assess Patient Satisfaction of Transitioning from Medicaid to Managed Care by Sickle Cell Patients in Hampton Roads, Virginia

Judy Anderson, MA
Sheila D. Miller, DSW

SUMMARY. Transition issues faced by the sickle cell patient who has a significant chronic illness or disability are many and often life threatening. The problems that are faced in transitioning from Medicaid to managed care are many that could hinder the process and patient satisfaction. Such problems during the transition periods could stem from interrupted health care services; improperly coordinated services; inappropriate intervention; and inappropriate or unfounded psychologically diagnosed cases (Blum, 1993). It is not known which health care programs are cost-effective and which are not. Nor is it known which health care program best meets the needs of patients with chronic illnesses or varying levels of severity; and it is not known if health status actually improves as a result of transitioning from one program to another.

What factors then impact the satisfaction levels in transitioning from Medicaid to managed care for sickle cell patients in Hampton Roads,

Judy Anderson is Executive Director, Sickle Cell Association, Inc. Norfolk, VA. Sheila D. Miller is Professor, Norfolk State University, Norfolk, VA.

[Haworth co-indexing entry note]: "A Study to Assess Patient Satisfaction of Transitioning from Medicaid to Managed Care by Sickle Cell Patients in Hampton Roads, Virginia." Anderson, Judy, and Sheila D. Miller. Co-published simultaneously in *Journal of Health & Social Policy* (The Haworth Press, Inc.) Vol. 16, No. 1/2, 2002, pp. 5-20; and: *Disability and the Black Community* (ed: Sheila D. Miller) The Haworth Press, Inc., 2002, pp. 5-20. Single or multiple copies of this article are available for a fee from The Haworth Document Delivery Service [1-800-HAWORTH, 9:00 a.m. - 5:00 p.m. (EST). E-mail address: docdelivery @haworthpress.com].

Virginia? This study looked at patient satisfaction with the transition from Medicaid to managed care as related to the cost of care, quality of care, and access to care. *[Article copies available for a fee from The Haworth Document Delivery Service: 1-800-HAWORTH. E-mail address: <docdelivery@ haworthpress.com> Website: <http://www.HaworthPress.com> © 2002 by The Haworth Press, Inc. All rights reserved.]*

KEYWORDS. Medicaid, managed care, cost of care, quality of care, access to care

INTRODUCTION

Medicaid was created in 1965 along with the Medicare program. It was essentially a grant program, jointly funded by the federal and state governments. The federal government pays just over 50 percent of the Medicaid bill, however that share varies from state to state (Califano, 1986). A major problem with Medicaid has been the definition of the medically needy by various states. Unfortunately, according to the Advisory Commission on Intergovernmental Relations, many states set the levels of need far below any reasonable standards of adequacy. This inequity creates a migration pull to areas with more generous benefits. The federal government does not impose uniform standards on the states (McTaggart and McTaggart, 1971). The Balanced Budget Act of 1997 was passed by Congress and included a number of significant health-related provisions. The Act had a major impact on the provision of financing of health care for Virginia's Medicare and Medicaid populations. It provided approximately $13 billion in Medicaid savings over five years and lowered the cost of Medicare for low-income beneficiaries by $1.5 billion over the same period (Joint Commission on Health Care, 1997).

Managed care has become the predominant system for the delivery of health care in the United States (Kovner, 1995). The driving force behind this growth in health care delivery is the belief that managing health care can also control health care costs. Although not directly attributable to legislative activity, the effect of the penetration of managed health care plans on the provision of genetic services cannot be overlooked. As a result, a basic transformation in the way service provision is organized, delivered, and, most importantly, financed is occurring. The driving force for the new order in health care delivery is the supreme position occupied by economic considerations in managed care plans (Cohen, 1996). Transition issues faced by the sickle cell patients with a significant chronic illness or disability are many and often life threatening. The findings in this research study addressed the issues of cost effectiveness, access to care, and quality of care as related to patient satisfaction with transitioning from Medicaid to a managed health care plan.

RESEARCH DESIGN

Data Collection Instrument

The data collection instrument was a non-standardized, 26 item, Patient Satisfaction Questionnaire. The questionnaire was created from a composite of the patient satisfaction survey questions used by Trigon Healthkeepers and the Sickle Cell Center at Grady Hospital in Atlanta, Georgia. (See Figures 1 and 2.) The instrument was printed on a one-sided sheet for ease of reading. The Likert scale was employed using the standardized response categories of poor, fair, good, very good and excellent.

One hundred participants were recruited to participate in the study. The participants were sickle cell disease patients. The participant names were randomly selected from the case files at the Sickle Cell Association and the Peninsula Association for Sickle Cell Anemia. Primary participants were adult sickle cell patients, 18 years of age and older who had Medicaid coverage before the transition to managed care plans. Another group were parents of sickle cell children who were identified from a large number of cases in the Agency files. The 100 participants were residents from throughout the Hampton Roads, Virginia area. Case files had 382 sickle cell patient names and addresses listed. The names were selected from every third draw on the listing.

The questionnaires on patient satisfaction were first administered through mailings. After the first two weeks of no returns, telephone calls and face-to-face interviews were made to insure that the participant understood the nature of the study and to gather more responses. Prior to administering the questionnaire on levels of satisfaction, a letter was sent to each participant with an explanation that the information being gathered was for statistical purposes only.

Variables

In this study there were three independent variables and one dependent variable. The three independent variables were cost of care, access to care and quality of care. The dependent variable was the level of satisfaction with the transition to managed care. The Patient Satisfaction Questionnaire addressed three exploratory research questions on: What was the level of satisfaction with cost of care? What was the level of satisfaction with access to care and what was the level of satisfaction with quality of care?

The biggest cost of managed care coverage for most consumers is the monthly premium. However, Medicaid-managed care participants did not have to pay the monthly premium. The participants may have co-payments for visits to the doctor's offices, for prescription drugs, and sometimes for emer-

FIGURE 1. Sickle Cell Acute Care: Frequency Over 52 Visits/Yr

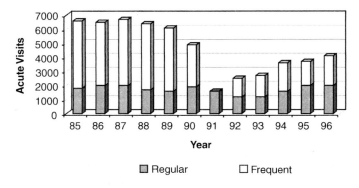

Sources: Comprehensive Sickle Cell Center (Atlanta), Grady Health System,
Emory University School of Medicine. Printed with Permission.

gency room care and hospitalization. Since sickle cell patients are frequent users of medical services, their perception of future changes was an important issue should their economic situation change and they needed to purchase medical insurance. A consideration in the questionnaire addressed the frequent visits of patients to the primary care physician. Sickle cell patients fall in the high-user category of medical services so there was a question about current experiences in paying for medical care.

Access to care is an indicator to be addressed. There are several kinds of access to care that are important to most consumers. The sickle cell patient experiencing a critical pain crisis will need to know how quickly they can get an appointment; what kind of treatment they will receive when they are really sick; or how quickly could they get an appointment for routine, non-urgent visits? How easily can they get through on the phone when they have urgent medical concerns? How long will they have to wait in the doctor's waiting rooms for scheduled appointments? These questions assessed the managed care participants' satisfaction with access to care and measured the satisfaction level with accessed appointments as well as how long a patient waited in the waiting room. This kind of information was most useful in the comparison of satisfaction from one variable to another.

Everyone wants high quality of health care. The questionnaire touched on how satisfied the patient was with the managed care plan selected since transitioning

FIGURE 2. Sickle Cell Center: Admissions per Total Patients

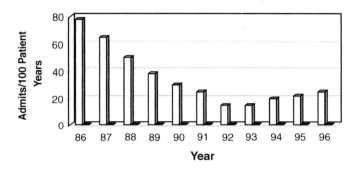

Sources: Comprehensive Sickle Cell Center (Atlanta), Grady Health System, Emory University School of Medicine. Printed with Permission.

from Medicaid services. It asked patients to rate their satisfaction with the technical skills of the medical personnel they saw; an explanation of what was done; the personal manner of the medical personnel seen; and the time spent with the medical personnel. Until recently, there had been no commonly accepted formula for satisfaction issues in health care quality; for the consumer it usually was more was better. More services, more technology and more expensive care were all thought to equal better quality of care. Medical experts now agree that this is not necessarily true. There are rapidly evolving new systems for measuring and reporting on health care quality based on what is appropriate and effective (National Committee for Quality Assurance, 1997). Measured responses focused on the patient's satisfaction with the overall managed care plan from the cost of care, the quality of care and with their ability to have easy access to care when they needed it.

Limitation of Study

The limitations of this study did not take into account that the questionnaire may be lost in the mail, and the two-week turn around time was lost for some returns thereby hindering the return rates on the instruments. Other limitations indicated that some patients had experienced health status deterioration as a result of repeated strokes or blindness and could not answer the questionnaire mailed. However, the volunteers were given orientation to give patients a face-to-face interview. The same amount of time, 15 minutes, was allowed for each interview session. Therefore no special treatment had to be given for administering the surveys. Other problems in collecting data resulted from patients moving and leaving no forwarding address or the forwarding period had expired in the post office. Volunteers tried to reach some of the patients by the last listed phone number and found that not all patients had transitioned to a managed care plan as had been suggested. Even though the number was small, two cases were found that had not made the transition but this did not hinder the completion of the study.

The delimitations of the study showed that the research did not seek to impact policy by determining which managed care plan is better than another plan. It was the intent of this research to assess the patient satisfaction with transitioning from the Medicaid program to a managed care plan. The patient needed to have some knowledge of both plans, Medicaid and Managed Care before answering the questionnaire.

The reality of such a study as this has the limits of comparative information from one plan to another. Since managed care plans are new for many Medicaid recipients, this study can serve as a baseline to the hope that ongoing studies will measure these factors over time. This will serve as a useful tool in the health care delivery field when referrals are needed for the chronically ill, sickle cell patients.

ANALYSIS OF DATA

Analysis of the Data

Literature review for statistical methods suggested that the use of multiple correlation and regression strategies would be the best treatment of the data collected (Babbie, 1989). The multiple regression models permit the inclusion of several predictor variables, which improves the predictive value of the model to explain variances in a criterion variable.

Data was tested through analyses of variance of the three sub-hypotheses. The statistical values generated from the statistical runs on the Statistical Package for the Social Sciences (SPSS) formed the basis upon which the significance of variable in the study was formed (Babbie, 1989). Based upon the proposed prediction model of patient satisfaction for the study, multiple correlation and regression were used.

Demographic Information

A total of 70 surveys were completed and returned, resulting in a 70 percent return rate. This is considerably higher than the typical return data (Babbie,

1989). Ages were evenly distributed, from a low of 4 to a high of 67. The mode ages were 22 and 29 years (8.9 percent each). Thirty-six percent of respondents were male and 64 percent were females. The majority (49.2 percent) indicated that high school was the highest level of education completed. Another 24.6 percent had completed elementary school, 23 percent had completed college, and 3.3 percent had completed some type of post-high school training.

Results of the data are presented as follows:

1. demographic information (city of residence, disease type, education level and household income);
2. correlation coefficients; and
3. standard multiple regression analysis.

The majority of respondents (36 percent) have household incomes greater than $15,000. Thirty-two percent (32%) have incomes less than $5,000; 20 percent have incomes between $5,001 and $10,000; and 12 percent have incomes between $10,001 and $15,000 as indicated in Figure 3.

Figure 4 showed that the majority of respondents (68.8 percent) suffered from Sickle Cell Anemia. Twenty-six (26%) suffered from Sickle C Disease, and 6 percent suffered from Sickle Thalassemia. These are all varying types of abnormal sickling diseases that have varying degrees of pain episodes. Sickle Cell Anemia is the most severe of the disease types. The majority of the respondents (31 percent) resided in Norfolk, Virginia. Twenty-three percent (23%) lived in Virginia Beach, 11 percent in Suffolk and 9 percent in Newport News, Virginia. The remainder resided in Hampton, Chesapeake, Smithfield, Portsmouth, Franklin and Waverly.

Satisfaction with Health Care Services

Respondents were most satisfied with the effectiveness of the care they received from their doctors, the overall health care visit to their doctors, and referrals to specialists. Over one-fourth of respondents (29.7 percent) rated effectiveness of care as excellent, as did 27.7 percent for satisfaction with overall office visits and 20 percent for referrals to specialists.

In contrast, based on ratings of poor, 10.9 percent expressed dissatisfaction with their experience in paying health care bills. Nine percent (9%) gave their health plan an overall rating of poor, and 7.7 percent rated emergency room and hospital care poor (Figure 5).

Correlation Coefficients

Satisfaction with health plans was significantly correlated ($p < .05$) with all variables excluding the condition of the waiting room. Emergency/hospital

FIGURE 3. Respondent's Household Income

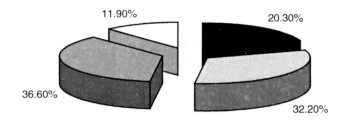

FIGURE 4. Respondent's Disease Type

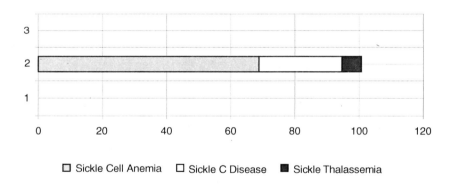

☐ Sickle Cell Anemia   ☐ Sickle C Disease   ■ Sickle Thalassemia

services and experience with paying was most strongly correlated with satisfaction (r = .694 and .695 respectively). The only inverse correlation with satisfaction with health care was with gender (r = −.325). This indicated that
male respondents were slightly more satisfied with their health care plans than
were female respondents.

Several other variables were also highly correlated with each other. Most
strongly associated was the relationship between time spent with health care
professionals and explanation of treatment procedure (r = .897). Time spent
with health care professionals was also highly correlated with the personal
manner of the professional staff (r = .880). Similarly, the personal manner of
the professional staff was highly correlated between satisfaction with explana-

FIGURE 5. Satisfaction with Health Care Services (Percentages)

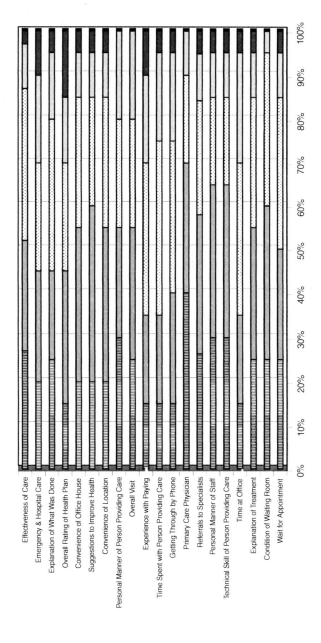

13

tion of treatment (r = .835) and effectiveness of care (r = .815). Finally, associations between ratings of primary care physician and effectiveness of care, as well as explanation of treatment and overall satisfaction with visits, are statistically significant at $p < .05$ (r = .885 and .865 respectively).

Ages, city of residence, gender, income and disease type are not significantly correlated with any variables in the study. A complete table of all significant relationships ($p < .05$) can be found in Table 1.

Discussion on Findings

The variables included in the analysis accounted for 90.5 percent of the variance in satisfaction with a health plan. Adjusted for the number of cases included in the analysis, this rate dropped significantly to 55.5 percent. Analysis of the data using the Statistical Package for Social Sciences (SPSS, Windows version 7.0) gives the multiple regression analysis and Analysis of Variance (ANOVA). Social Research on findings identifies the higher the beta weight or standardized regression coefficients, the greater the relative effect of the particular predictor variable on the dependent variable when all the other variables are constant (Babbie, 1989). The independent variables with the highest beta weight included emergency and hospital care, suggestions to improve health; rating of primary physician and length of wait for an appointment had the highest beta weight as significant predictor variables (Table 2).

Statistical Package for Social Sciences (SPSS) runs the series mean in all cases, which has missing data. Basically, any missing data was treated as the average response for the population sampled. As a result, 70 surveys were returned and analyzed. Twenty-eight surveys contained missing data on one or more of the variables. This would indicate a skew in the data used for analysis (Babbie, 1989). However, analysis of the demographic information indicated an even distribution for ages, household income, and highest level of school attainment, type of disease and city residence. Therefore, it was reasonable to speculate that responses on the completed surveys were representative of responses on those with missing data.

It is recommended that when conducting multiple regressions, there should be a minimum of five cases for each independent variable. In the present analysis, a total of 125 cases can decrease the dispersion of variable scores, thereby understating the relationships between variables. Data elements were highly correlated and could have impacted the outcome of the regression analysis (Tabachnick and Fidell, 1989). As indicated in the discussion of correlation coefficients and the accompanying correlation matrix, many of the survey elements were highly correlated ($p > .70$). Multicolinearity can be determined by examination of the Tolerance values in the regression Table 3 (Kazmier,

TABLE 1. Significant (p < .05) Correlation Coefficients

	Effective	Emerg	Explain	Gender	House	Improve	Location	Manner	Overall	Paying	Person	Phone	Primary	Refer	Staff	Techskl	Time	Trtmt	Watrm	Waitme
Healthplan	.511	.694	.459	-.325	-.584	.520	.504	.501	.449	.656	.474	.444	.511	.572	.432	.560	.516	.551	—	.485
Effective		.558	.771	—	.673	.773	.626	.815	.799	.417	.590	.379	.885	.776	.630	.609	.498	.785	.534	.616
Emerg/hosp			.547	-.291	.538	.638	.507	.543	.529	.799	.500	.513	.476	.505	.464	.511	.577	.501	.312	.438
Explan					.682	.722	.673	.835	.865	.406	.897	.379	.771	.636	.472	.764	.625	.718	.462	.728
House						.628	.624	.651	.645	.518	.683	.651	.592	.624	.687	.698	.746	.763	.746	.702
Improve							.513	.774	.686	.495	.621	.545	.737	.652	.537	.628	.522	.691	.399	.702
Location								.533	.658	.490	.694	.481	.633	.605	.619	.544	.498	.662	.639	.448
Manner									.840	.425	.713	.356	.755	.656	.571	.811	.532	.699	.452	.713
Overall										.344	.880	.450	.713	.612	.566	.728	.664	.723	.452	.671
Paying											.449	.390	.364	.364	.479	.320	.485	.481	.319	.671
Person												.432	.644	.599	.531	.643	.747	.799	.496	.297
Phone													.281	.491	.458	.520	.646	.489	.543	.728
Primary														.804	.580	.596	.411	.754	.494	.573
Referral															.534	.675	.440	.793	.405	.539
Staff																.540	.577	.634	.761	.650
Techskill																	.580	.644	.457	.535
Time																		.617	.539	.775
Treatment																			.567	.640
Waitroom																				.669

15

TABLE 2. Patient Satisfaction with Cost of Care, Access to Care, Quality of Care

Model 1	Unstandardized Coefficients		Standardized Coefficients	t	Sig.
	B	Std. Error	Beta		
Getting Through by Phone	−9.4E-02	.203	−.091	−.465	.644
Rate Primary Care	.340	.302	.283	1.124	.267
Physician Referrals to Specialist	5.6E-02	.206	.054	.269	.789
Highest Grade Completed	−.127	.190	−.082	−.667	.508
Personal Manner of Staff	.160	.200	.139	.801	.427
Technical Skill of Person	.115	.210	.106	.546	.588
Length of Time at Office	.185	.230	.176	.805	.425
Explanation about Treatment	1.0E-02	.217	.009	.046	.963
Condition of Waiting Room	−9.1E-02	.228	−.069	−.400	.691
Length of Wait for Appointment	.328	.238	.298	1.377	.176
(Constant)	.783	1.106		.708	.483
Age	1.8E-02	.013	.169	1.417	.163
City of Residence	−.107	.075	−.190	−1.428	.160
Type of Disease	−9.9E-02	.212	−.054	−.468	.642
Effectiveness of Care	−.310	.309	−.282	−1.002	.322
Emergency and Hospital Care	.257	.178	.282	1.444	.156
Explanation of What Was Done	−.126	.279	−.121	−.452	.653
Gender	−9.7E-02	.264	−.041	−.368	.714
Convenience of Office House	4.6E-02	.246	.041	.185	.854
Suggestions to Improve Health	.308	.209	.299	1.476	.147
Household Income	−.138	.128	−.145	−1.080	.265
Convenience of Location	−.117	.194	−.114	−.606	.548
Personal Manner of Person	−.164	.247	−.145	−.663	.511
Visit Overall	8.0E-02	.311	.067	.256	.799
Experience w/Paying	.127	.184	.133	.688	.495
Time Spent with Person	−.124	.257	−.116	−.484	.631

Model	Sum of Squares	df	Mean Square	F	Sig.
2 Regression	55.584	25	2.222	2.796	.001[b]
Residual	34.966	44	.795		
Total	90.515	69			

a. Dependent Variable: Patient Satisfaction
b. Independent Variables: (Constant), Length of Wait for Appointment, Gender, Highest Grade Completed, Type of Disease, Age, Household Income, Experience w/Paying, City of Residence, Rate Primary Care Physician, Condition of Waiting Room, Personal Manner of Person, Getting Through by Phone, Time Spent with Person, Personal Manner of Staff, Explanation about Treatment, Convenience of Location, Referrals to Specialists, Emergency and Hospital Care, Technical Skill of Person, Suggestions to Improve Health, Convenience of Office House, Length of Time at Office, Visit Overall, Explanation of What Was Done, Effectiveness of Care.

1988). The independent variables in Table 3 were highly correlated with one another for the multiple regression analysis. Therefore the partial (or net) regression coefficients are unreliable in siginificance and definitive meaning. A tolerance value less than $1-R^2$ (.18) indicated that a variable was highly correlated with at least one other independent variable in the analysis. Effectiveness of care, Explanation of Treatment, Improvement in Health, Manner of Health Care Professional, Overall Rating of Visit, Time Spent with Person Providing Care, Referral to Specialists, and Length of Wait for Appointment all have very low tolerance values. These variables also have high correlation coefficients in the coefficient matrix.

High correlation can be expected with these variables due to the fact that the measure of one or two constructs was found for either access to care or quality of care. All variables were included in the survey instrument. Future research should be conducted to determine which combination of survey questions could be utilized to best predict patient satisfaction with health plans.

Regression Analysis

A standard multiple regressions was performed between satisfaction with health plan as the dependent variable collected on the survey instrument and correlated with the independent variables. Analysis was performed using SPSS version 6.1 for Windows (Student Version). Table 3 displays the non-standardized regression coefficients (B), the standard error of regression coefficients (SE B), tolerance values, t-values and significance, as well as R, R^2 and adjusted R^2.

The coefficients indicated the proportion of variance in the dependent variable, patient satisfaction, which is statistically accounted for by the knowledge of the three independent variables: cost of care, access to care and quality of care. Consideration of the coefficient of multiple-determination included in the computer output and the interpretation of the coefficient provided an analysis model for this study.

CONCLUSIONS

This study revealed that there was high correlation between the independent variables. The highest correlations among variables were for effectiveness of care, explanation of treatment, improvement in health, manner of health care professional, overall rating of visit, time spent with person providing care, referrals to specialist, and length of wait for appointment. These variables also showed the lowest tolerance values among the patients surveyed.

TABLE 3

Multiple R   .90687
R Square   .82242
Adjusted R Squarre .54495   F = 2.96398   Sig. F. = .0138

Variable	B	SE B	Tolerance	T	Sig. T
Age	.009076	.016217	.568493	.560	.5835
City	−.159334	.099289	.369601	−1.605	.1281
Disease	.037610	.313661	.486021	.120	.9060
Effective	.651576	.535500	.047735	1.217	.2413
Emerg.	.175588	.278677	.124119	.630	.5375
Explain	−.949329	.648313	.029346	−1.464	.1625
Gender	−532071	.337666	.588736	−1.576	.1347
House	.631937	.422033	.107976	1.497	.1538
Improve	.055311	.369746	.097035	.150	.8830
Location	.242053	.309335	.132590	.782	.4454
Manner	−.101954	.488149	.066245	−.209	.8372
Overall	−742150	.664024	.039094	−1.118	.2802
Paying	.034599	.305877	.116225	.113	.9113
Person	1.00705	.774088	.019162	1.301	.2117
Phone	.199462	.241764	.124779	.584	.5676
Primary	.315364	.472499	.074452	.667	.5140
Referral	−.255584	.352369	.095784	−.725	.4787
School	−.277626	.233311	.517139	−1.190	.2514
Staff	.014633	.366258	.151175	.040	.9686
Techskil	.787205	.398063	.082313	1.978	.0565
Time	−.093597	.265968	.158919	−.352	.7295
Treatmt	−.580037	.451864	.088065	−1.284	.2175
Waitroom	−.719151	.434802	.118736	−1.654	.1176
Waittime	−.026507	.489325	.073257	−.054	.9575
(Constant)	3.692212	1.5471494		2.395	.0292

The sickle cell patient has a lifetime of required medical care and frequent hospitalizations. Whether joining a managed care plan is by choice or the only choice, sickle cell patients should be very clear in their minds what level of care they will receive under a particular plan. Many persons with the disease still have to deal with the lack of knowledge and understanding about the disease from providers and the public. The ability to choose from among the many managed care plan doctors was very important to sickle cell patients as well as being able to get care at a local hospital if they are very sick. Choosing the right health care plan can seem like an overwhelming task especially if you have a chronic illness that requires certain specialties to treat the complicating manifestations of the disease. For sickle cell disease as with any chronic illness patients need to develop short and long-term psychological and social skills necessary to successfully navigate the medical and social systems in which they function (LePontis, Hurtig, and Viera, 1986).

This study did not determine a significant degree of patient satisfaction with transitioning from Medicaid to a managed care plan. The three priority areas of cost of care, access to care and quality of care were not determined as significant patient satisfaction variables.

Future research should be conducted to determine which combination of variables directly impacts patient satisfaction with a specific managed care plan. A clear understanding is essential if health care is to remain viable in the changing health care system. Managed care plans are relatively new in the health care industry. A follow-up study in the future would be necessary to determine if a comparative analysis can show any significance of change in patient satisfaction and transition issues over time. Management of the at-risk sickle cell population is an important aspect of the health care market that has implications for future impact studies on proposed health care reform and managed care systems.

REFERENCES

Annual Report, Culver City, CA: (1977) Sickle Cell Disease Association of America, Inc.

Babbie, E. (1989). *The Practice of Social Research*, p. 63, 238-242. Belmont: Wadsworth Publishing Company.

Blum, Robert William. (1993) *Transition from Child Centered to Adult Health Care Systems for Adolescents with Chronic Conditions*, p. 570. New York: Elsevier Science Publishing Company.

Califano, Jr., Joseph. (1986) *America's Health Care Revolution: Who Lives? Who Dies? Who Pays?*, pp. 3-10, 151. New York: Random House.

Cohen, M. (1996) The Impact of the Current Legislative Climate on Genetic Services, *Genetic Services: Developing Guidelines for the Public Health*, p. 142. Atlanta: The Council of Regional Networks for Genetic Services.

Eckman, James R. and Allan F. Platt. (1991) *Problem Oriented Management of Sickle Cell Syndromes*, pp. 3-6. Atlanta: Grady Hospital Department of Genetics.

Joint Commission on Health Care. (1997) *Study of the Indigent/Uninsured Phase III*. Richmond: Joint Commission on Health Care.

Kazmier, Leonard. (1988) *Business Statistics and Computer Applications*, p. 266. New York: McGraw-Hill, Inc.

Kovner, A. (1995) *Health Care Delivery in the United States*, p. 122. New York: Springer Publishing Company.

LePontis, J. A., L. Hurtig and C. T. Viera. (1986) "Adolescents with Sickle Cell Disease: Developmental Issues," *Sickle Cell Disease: Psychological and Psychosocial Issues*, pp. 75-83. Chicago: University of Illinois Press.

McTaggart, Aubrey and Lorna M. McTaggart. (1971) *The Health Care Dilemma*, p. 267. Boston: Allyn and Bacon, Inc.

National Committee for Quality Assurance Report. (1997) Washington, DC.

Stoline, Anne, MD. (1988) "From 1979 to Present: The Increasing Cost of Health Care," *The New Medical Market*, pp. 107-108. Baltimore: The Johns Hopkins University Press.

Tabachnick, B. and L. Fidell. (1989) *Using Multivariate Statistics*, pp. 123-189. New York: Harper Collins Publisher.

Help-Seeking and Risk-Taking Behavior Among Black Street Youth: Implications for HIV/AIDS Prevention and Social Policy

Cudore L. Snell, PhD

SUMMARY. This article explores and analyzes the help-seeking and risk-taking behavior of Black urban street youth in Washington, DC, USA and Cape Town, South Africa. The target population of 100 youths came from the streets of Washington, DC and Cape Town, South Africa. Structured face-to-face interviews and direct observation of informal and formal settings where youths congregated were used to gather data. Major findings indicate that the majority received high levels of support from families and friends. In terms of formal systems, social and mental health services are viewed as much less accessible or useful. Youths were knowledgeable about HIV/AIDS but did not translate this into safer sexual practices. Implications for health and social policy are outlined. *[Article copies available for a fee from The Haworth Document Delivery Service: 1-800-HAWORTH. E-mail address: <docdelivery@haworthpress.com> Website: <http://www.HaworthPress.com> © 2002 by The Haworth Press, Inc. All rights reserved.]*

KEYWORDS. Street youth, help-seeking, risk-taking, HIV/AIDS prevention, South Africa, United States of America

Dr. Cudore L. Snell is an Associate Professor in the School of Social Work, and Associate Dean for Academic Affairs at Howard University, Washington, DC.

[Haworth co-indexing entry note]: "Help-Seeking and Risk-Taking Behavior Among Black Street Youth: Implications for HIV/AIDS Prevention and Social Policy." Snell, Cudore, L. Co-published simultaneously in *Journal of Health & Social Policy* (The Haworth Press, Inc.) Vol. 16, No. 1/2, 2002, pp. 21-32; and: *Disability and the Black Community* (ed: Sheila D. Miller) The Haworth Press, Inc., 2002, pp. 21-32. Single or multiple copies of this article are available for a fee from The Haworth Document Delivery Service [1-800-HAWORTH, 9:00 a.m. - 5:00 p.m. (EST). E-mail address: docdelivery@haworthpress.com].

http://www.haworthpress.com/store/product.asp?sku=J045
10.1300/J045v16n01_03

The developmental stages of adolescence and early adulthood are characterized by a variety of tasks, including physical maturation, membership in a peer group, autonomy from parents, sexual relationships and gender identity. These can involve experimentation, conflict, tension and alienation and almost certainly change and experiences for new challenges and opportunities. There is no uniformity about the definition of youth. Theorists have conceptualized youth in many different ways. Some have defined youth as the stage between adolescence and adulthood (Thom, 1991) and others used the term synonymously with those of "teenager" and "adolescent," referring to someone between childhood and adulthood (Chalke, 1987). The definitions offered by Bundy (1992) and Riordan (1992) fit the sample used in this study and were therefore accepted. Their definition included adolescents, post-adolescents and young adults between the ages of approximately 13 and 29 or 30 years of age.

Youths in general, are more prone to sexual experimentation and other risk-taking behaviors than other age groups. While this may be true, it is also important to note that this age group may be the least likely to seek or accept help unless certain developmental aspects are taken into consideration. Street youths on the other hand, are extremely vulnerable to the personal and social risks from being on the streets no matter where in the world they find themselves.

Health is a complex and multi-dimensional concept and may be defined in three main ways: in a negative or less proactive way as the absence of illness; in a functional way, as the ability to cope; or in a comprehensive way defined as "a state of complete physical, psychological and social well-being" (Blackburn, 1991). It is this last definition which incorporates a broad view of health encompassing both social and mental health and provides a useful context within which to understand the lives and risks of street youths (Morse, Simon & Burchfiel, 1999). This knowledge is critical to the design of effective prevention and intervention efforts aimed at arresting future HIV transmission or reducing HIV risk.

This article explores help-seeking and risk-taking behaviors in two samples of Black street youths from Washington, DC, USA and Cape Town, South Africa. Implications for intervention and policy are offered. This study is part of a larger one done on help-seeking behavior of street youths (Snell, 1995).

As an overall part of this inquiry, the social support systems of street youths are identified and described. "Help-seeking" is defined as those actions aimed at problem-solving through requesting advice and/or material and emotional assistance from formal and informal resources. Formal resources consist of social agencies, programs and professionals, while informal sources included friends, family and peers (Barth, 1983; Gary, Leashore, Howard & Buckner-Dowell, 1983; Gottlieb, 1980, 1981; Gourash, 1978; Israel, 1985).

The research specifically addressed the following questions:

1. Who seeks help?
2. What kind of help is sought?
3. What social supports exist for street youths and what role do these systems play in help-seeking behavior?
4. What are the levels of HIV/AIDS knowledge, attitudes and behavior among Black street youths in the USA and South Africa?

There continues to be a dearth in the social science literature concerning the resilience of Black youths and their families. Most of the studies tend to focus on their problems and disconnection from family. Clearly absent from most of the literature is any reference to their strengths, particularly their ability to seek and receive both formal and informal assistance (Snell, 1995). The dominant research ideology provides in essence a disease model of youth, justifying policies focused on individual treatment. Policies pressure families to adhere to specific behavioral changes rather than promote social systemic changes which could strengthen prevention efforts through multi-modal, multi-sectoral and private-public partnerships (Akukwe, 2001; Pfeffer, 1997).

The most recent statistics are alarming and indicate the urgent and pressing needs for service providers and policy makers to intervene. A survey of 2,942 gay men ages 23 to 29 conducted in six cities from 1998 to 2000 found that 4.4% were becoming infected with HIV each year. The pace of new infections, varied greatlty by race and ethnicity. It was 2.5% among Whites, 3.5% among Hispanics and 14.7% among Blacks. The survey showed that 32% of young Black gays were already infected as were 14% of Hispanics and 7% of Whites. The implications for developing effective prevention messages are clear (CDC, 2000).

A recent White House report estimated that one in four new seroconversions for HIV is among youths aged 13 to 20 (Fleming, 1996). Fully two-thirds of adolescents in the United States of America have had sexual intercourse by age 19, although less than 10% report regular condom use (Flora & Thoresen, 1989). A marker of a youth being at high risk for HIV is that sexually active adolescents have the highest rates of sexually transmitted diseases of all age groups (DiClemente, 1992; Flisher, 1993; Hein, 1993; Perry & Sieving, 1991; Walters, 1999). If one takes into account the average 10 to 11 year lag between initial infection and AIDS diagnosis, when considering that AIDS is the leading cause of death among 25 to 44 year olds in the US, it is also evident that many adults become HIV positive during adolescence and young adulthood (CDC, 1996). Young people in the US and in South Africa are clearly at risk for HIV/AIDS (Walters, 1999; Kral, Molnar, Booth & Watters, 1997; Flisher, 1993; Swart-Kruger & Richter, 1997). This is even more alarming when considering that street youths have seroprevalence rates 10-25 times higher than other groups of adolescents (Sondheimer, 1992; Sugerman et al., 1991; Walters,

1999). Runaway and homeless youths in South Africa and in the United States have been neglected and excluded from major studies on HIV/AIDS (Rotheram-Borus, Feldman, Rosario et al., 1994).

METHODS

A survey design with an informal semi-structured interview schedule was the chief method used to obtain exploratory descriptive-analytic data. The target populations consisted of non-random, convenience samples of 70 street youths in Washington, DC, USA and 30 in Cape Town, South Africa who sought out the services of private non-profit social service agencies in large urban environments. Face-to-face interviews were conducted in booths during colder weather, at fast food eating places in the United States of America. One residential facility and an alternative school setting in South Africa served as sites for collecting data. In warmer weather, interviews were conducted in nearby parks where the youths congregated. Snowball sampling was used to counter the potential difficulty of reaching non-captive subjects and to reduce the levels of mistrust and hostility. Interviews were conducted by the researcher and a second trained interviewer in each country.

Both quantitative and qualitative items were used for this research. The personal interview schedule consisting of open-ended as well as forced-choice, Likert type questions was constructed and modified from the Social Support Behaviors Scale (SS-B) (Vaux, Riedel & Stewart, 1987). Items were taken from the National Survey of Black Americans (NSBA) which was conducted at the University of Michigan in 1970-1980. These items were culturally appropriate for use with Black South African youth.

The interview schedule gathered information on demographic and background characteristics such as age, race, years of school completed, employment status, living arrangements, and level of satisfaction with life. Help-seeking and risk-taking behaviors were also assessed as well as knowledge and safer sexual practices regarding HIV/AIDS.

RESULTS

The results are presented to answer the research questions posed earlier: Who seeks help? What kind of help is sought? What social support systems exist for street youths and what role do these systems play in help-seeking behavior? What are the levels of knowledge of HIV/AIDS, attitudes and behavior among Black street youths in the United States of America and South Africa?

Who Seeks Help?

A socio-demographic profile of the youths best describes the help-seekers in this study. In the United States, the mean age of the respondents was 22 years, with a range of 14 to 34. The sample was almost evenly distributed as to race: white (50%) and African American (46%). Half of the subjects were born in the South and claimed Southern Baptist as their religious affiliation. More than half of the subjects (57%) had a high school education. More than half of the subjects (58%) were currently living somewhere on a short-term basis. A third of them had been raised by their mothers alone, another third by two parents and a third by other relatives. Most of them had jobs ranging from non-technical such as courier, hospital worker, or clerk; to technical jobs such as word processor, landscaper, or air conditioning repairman. More than 60% of the subjects worked either full-time or part-time.

The majority (89%) reported that they were worried about the following in order of importance: AIDS and physical danger; the future; and personal relationships. While the majority expressed worries, almost all (97%) also reported that they had "fun" times, enjoyed mostly with close friends. Activities engaged in included: getting high, playing sports, hanging out at malls, partying, and sex. The majority (62%) reported being satisfied with life in general.

There were several contrasts and fewer similarities in the Cape Town, South Africa sample. Youths ranged in age from 7 to 18 years with the majority between 12 and 14 years, with a mean age of 13 years. Similar findings were reported by researchers in South Africa and elsewhere (Le Roux, 1996; Raffaelli, 1997; Richter, 1991; Scharff, Powell & Thomas, 1986; Swart-Kruger & Richter, 1997). The sample was all Black. There are virtually no white street youths. Most (95%) of the subjects were born in the Cape Town urban areas. None of the subjects had completed high school; 90% attended an alternative grade school for homeless and runaway youth. Eighty-five percent were living with extended family on a short-term basis ranging in length from one week to a few months. Most of them were raised by grandmothers and aunts. Almost all of the street youths (9%) expressed that they worried about the following in order of seriousness: personal relationships, usually other siblings and mothers; basic needs such as food and shelter; physical danger and AIDS. This was in reverse order from the US sample. There was some income from sexual activity ranging from about $3 to $25. Ninety-five percent had "unrealistic" aspirations for future occupations like becoming lawyers, air stewards, doctors and teachers.

What Kind of Help is Sought?

Subjects in the United States' sample sought help from informal sources (friends, family, and peers) as well as from formal sources (social agencies and professionals). The majority (63%) reported high levels of current emotional support from family, when and if they needed it, despite their emotional and geographic distances from biological parents and siblings. Fifty-seven percent reported having received high levels of material support from their families. This finding is consistent with previous studies reporting that the family is usually the first line of support for Blacks before professional help is sought (Gary et al., 1983; McAdoo, 1981). The support African American families provide for family members has been well documented (Billingsley, 1968; English, 1974; Hill, 1971; McAdoo, 1981). In line with this, more African American street male youths (42%) learned about places to go for help from their families compared to white street male youths (13%). More African American males (68%) were reluctant to seek help from traditional helping sources such as employment agencies, or alcoholics/narcotics anonymous compared to white males (43%). Also, African American and white males differed in relation to the reasons they offered for not seeking help from various traditional sources. For the African American youths, solving one's own problems or at least keeping it in the family and among friends, seemed to be paramount. They viewed this not in a pathological way, but as providing many strengths that help them withstand oppression in a racist society (See, 1986). African American youths were reluctant to admit they need help and did not wish to be perceived as needing help, seeing such need as a sign of personal weakness or failure. The fear of what others may think of them was expressed by 64% of African American youths. White males, on the other hand, were more likely (65%) to cite lack of money as a major deterrent to seeking help, for example, not having the money for transportation. Whether the two populations are saying the same thing in different ways would be interesting to explore in relation to norms for African American and white male socialization.

These findings are consistent with scholars who found that African American male youths in particular, are reluctant to seek help from mental health service professionals because of stigmas attached to seeking help. Mainstream traditional agencies seem not to reach African American males effectively (Gary et al., 1983; Gibbs, 1988). Informants were less likely to rely on friends for material support. Fifty-seven percent indicated they had received low levels of support from their friends.

The majority (61%) reported that they would, if necessary, seek help from a hospital emergency room, medical clinic, minister or lawyer. This finding, which indicates an overall pattern of seeking formal assistance, is an appropriate response to the kinds of problems for which they need help (Chatters & Taylor, 1989). A minority (39%) indicated that they would seek help from a social service or welfare agency, mental health center, police, alcoholics/narcotics anonymous, or a private therapist.

Respondents (85%) in the South African sample were more likely to seek help from informal sources (friends, family and peers) and less likely (87%) to seek help from formal sources (social agencies and professionals). The majority reported low levels of emotional support (72%) and material assistance (65%) from family. Unlike the United States sample, subjects from South Africa were more likely to rely on friends and peers for material needs (food, toiletries, money and shelter). Seventy-six percent indicated they had received high levels of support from their friends. The majority (87%) reported that they would not seek help from an emergency room, medical clinic, minister or lawyer. This was also true for 92% in terms of seeking help from a social service or welfare agency, mental health center, police, alcoholics/narcotics anonymous, or a private therapist. These services were limited and not part of their regular lives.

What Social Support Systems Does This Population Use?

Respondents in the USA found forms of help through friends (34%) and family (29%), advertisements (20%), professionals (10%), and through themselves (3%). The majority (91%) would return for help to the person they had gone to in the past if they needed to. They would also refer friends and family to the same source. Most of the respondents (87%) who have used formal services expressed satisfaction with the help they have received from social workers, counselors, doctors, lawyers, or ministers.

What is notable, is the reluctance to use local shelters despite the fact that the majority reported their willingness to seek help from a wide range of formal and informal social support systems. Reasons included: overcrowding, lack of privacy, concerns about cleanliness and security, feelings of humiliation, and restrictions on other regular activities.

In contrast, youths in South Africa had more limited access to a variety of sources such as friends, ads, and professionals to find forms of help for themselves. South Africa youths used teachers and each other exclusively. Youths in South Africa are also reluctant to use shelters for similar reasons, as in the US population, and added violence and rape to their list of reasons for not using shelters.

What Are the Levels of HIV/AIDS Knowledge, Attitudes and Behavior Among Black Street Youths?

Street youths, because of their activities placing themselves at risk, are extremely vulnerable to exposure to HIV. A striking set of findings indicates that while 81% report worrying about AIDS and 83% had someone they could confide in about AIDS, only 47% reported feeling at risk regarding AIDS; 40% did not think they were at risk, and 13% did not know their risk status. Eighty-five percent of the Black males reported not using condoms during oral-genital activity and 50% of the white males indicated that they did not use a condom during oral-genital activity.

Despite the limited use of condoms, many of the subjects reported a change or changes in sexual habits due to AIDS. For example, 89% of the white males and 55% of the Black males reported that they had changed their sexual habits due to the AIDS problem. However, current data show an increase in more risky sexual behavior which may be due to effective medicines and treatments for HIV/AIDS.

Different items were constructed and modified for cultural, cognitive and chronological appropriateness to the South African sample. Most of the youth had heard of AIDS from their teachers at school, knew it was an incurable disease and believed condoms to be effective. More than 60% did not know what it is and worried about AIDS. There was some lack of knowledge about the causes, symptomatology and transmission of AIDS. For example, one 15-year-old said: "you get it from sleeping with someone without a condom and three days later you get AIDS." There was also confusion about AIDS and other sexually transmitted diseases. There were perceptions that AIDS happened to "other" people, dirty people. It was something you "got" by associating with "immoral "persons.

Sixty-five percent of the youth reported that one could not get AIDS from a healthy looking person, and that one could tell from appearance if someone was HIV positive or had AIDS. Subjects described people with AIDS as gaunt-looking and who had sores on their genitals. AIDS was something to be scared of, clearly identifiable and unusual. Different standards of caring towards persons with HIV/AIDS were reported. If someone they did not know had AIDS, blame, anger and unconcern were expressed, whereas if it was someone they knew, empathic responses were shared. Similar findings were reported by scholars doing research on South African street youths (Swart-Kruger & Richter, 1997).

Other risk behaviors such as smoking cigarettes, drinking alcohol, using marijuana and sniffing glue were identified. All of the subjects participated in these behaviors. For this sample, there was an early onset of smoking cigarettes at an average age of 10 years which continued on a daily basis. The youngest age of onset for alcohol use was 10, with an average age of 14 years, and most drinking occurring over week-ends in the form of beer and wine. Using marijuana occurred on week-ends as well at the average age of 15 years. Most of the younger subjects reported sniffing glue.

IMPLICATIONS

It is clear that education programs aimed at increasing knowledge of HIV prevention and transmission are not sufficient, in and of themselves, to result in any serious reduction of HIV-related risk behavior (Booth, Zhang & Kwiatkowski, 1999). While preventative educational programs can effectively reduce risky behaviors among street youths, other options need to be explored as well (Rotheram-Borus, Lee, Murphy et al., 2001; Rotheram-Borus, O'Keefe, Kracker & Foo, 2001; Walters, 1999). What then are the implications of the data for HIV prevention and intervention health policy?

Health promotion and risk reduction services, according to the CDC, should occur at individual, group, and community levels (CDC, 1995). It should also reflect the local realities and culture wherein street youths and their families find themselves (Akukwe, 2001; Anarfi & Antwi, 1995; Smit & Liebenberg, 2000; Sorensen, Lopez & Anderson, 2001). Particularly recommended are the durable partnerships between government institutions, the business sector and community-based organizations; implementing outreach services in high-risk neighborhoods (Akukwe, 2001; Dryfoos, 1990). Especially relevant to South Africa, based on the research findings, would include reforms in the public schools and teacher support to address HIV/AIDS education as well as ways to address the myriad of accompanying social issues street youths face. Schools could serve as information and support centers since for many youth, these may be the only sources of consistent and reliable knowledge bases. In addition, given the medical and social consequences of HIV/AIDS, programs should include a medical doctor, a nurse, a psychologist, a counsellor and a social worker to assist in addressing the comprehensive needs of youths (Anarfi & Antwi, 1995; Goodridge & Capitman, 2000). Peer involvement, individual and group counselling were indicated as needs and effective methods to address HIV/AIDS and sexual concerns with youths which could be accommodated in school settings (CDC, 2000; Anarfi & Antwi, 1995; Gorgen, Yansane, Marx & Millimounou, 1998; Newman, 1999; Walters, 1999). Dryfoos (1990) recommends targeting high-risk neighborhoods and school districts rather than individuals given limited funding sources.

Findings suggest that effective shelter provision could enhance HIV/AIDS prevention messages to street youths. Youths in the United States and South Africa were reluctant to use shelters because of danger, stigma and restrictive policies. Addressing the issues of safety, restrictive policies and demystifying help-seeking, would facilitate their use of shelters. Similar findings were also documented in a study of runaway and homeless youths in California (Pennbridge, Yates, David et al., 1990). In South Africa, accessibility to shelters in the communities from which street youths come, are needed. In shelter settings, their health, mental health, economic, employment and housing needs can be addressed comprehensively. While Black youths in both the United States and South Africa face poverty and economic deprivation, addressing these needs are particularly urgent to youths in South Africa, vulnerable and susceptible to the resulting conditions of apartheid and urbanization.

Tackling unemployment, poverty, drug abuse and child abuse and neglect could advance a better quality of life for youths and their families, thus preventing the attraction and risks of the street. HIV risk-reduction interventions must also take into consideration the causes of homelessness, and individual factors such as the effects of sexual orientation, identity and ethnicity (Walters, 1999). Intervention programs and public policy that simultaneously target the psychological, economic and social needs of street youths and their families are essential to the success of any risk reduction program.

REFERENCES

Akukwe, C. (2001). The need for an urban HIV/AIDS policy in the United States. *Journal of Health and Social Policy, 12* (3), 1-15.

Barth, R. (1983). Social support networks in services for adolescents and their families. In Whittaker, J., and Garbarino, J. (Eds.). *Social support networks: Informal helping in the human services.* (299-330). New York: Aldine Publishing company

Billingsley, A. (1968). *Black families in white America.* Englewood Cliffs, NJ: Prentice-Hall.

Blackburn, C. (1991). *Poverty and health: Working with families.* Philadelphia, PA: Open University Press.

Bundy, C. (1992). Introduction. In Everatt, D. & Sisulu, E. (Eds.). *Black youth in crisis: Facing the future.* Braamfontein: Raven Press.

Chalke, S. (1987). *The complete youth manual* (Volume1). Eastbourne: Kingsway Publications.

Chatters, L. and Taylor, R. (1989). Life problems and coping strategies of older black adults. *Social Work, 34* (4), 313-319.

DiClemente, R. (1992). Epidemiology of AIDS/HIV seroprevalence and HIV incidence among adolescents. *Journal of School Health, 62,* 325-330.

Dryfoos, J. (1990). *Adolescents at risk.* New York & Oxford: Oxford University Press.

English, R. (1974). Beyond pathology: Research and theoretical perspectives on black families. In Gary, L. (Ed.) *Social research and the black community.* Washington, DC: Institute for Urban Affairs and Research, Howard University.

Fleming, P. (1996). *Youth and AIDS: A White House report.* Washington, DC: U.S. Government Printing Office.

Flisher, A. (1993). Risk-taking behaviour of Cape Peninsula high-school students: Part VIII. Sexual behaviour. *South African Medical Journal, 83,* 495-497.

Flora, J. and Thoresen, C. (1989). Reducing the risk of AIDS in adolescents. *American Psychologist, 43*(11), 965-970.

Gary, L., Leashore, B., Howard, C., and Buckner-Dowell, R. (1983). *Help-seeking behavior among black males (Final Report).* Washington, DC: Howard University, Institute for Urban Affairs and Research.

Gibbs, J. (1988). Black adolescents and youth: An endangered species. *American Journal of Orthopsychiatry, 54,* 6-22.

Gibbs, J. (1998). High-risk behaviors in African American youth: Conceptual and methodological issues in research. In Mcloyd, V. and Steinberg, L. (Eds.). *Studying minority adolescents.* Mahwah, NJ: Lawrence Erlbaum Associates, Inc.

Goodridge, L. and Capitman, J. (2000). Adolescents at risk for HIV infection. In Lynch, V. (Ed.). *HIV/AIDS at year 2000.* Boston, MA: Allyn & Bacon.

Gorgen, R., Yansane, M., Marx, M., and Millimounou, D. (1998). Sexual behavior and attitudes among unmarried urban youths in Guinea. *International Family Planning Perspectives, 24* (2), 65-71.

Gottlieb, B. (1980). *Social networks and the utilization of preventive mental health services.* Beverly Hills, CA: Sage Publications.

Gourash, N. (1981). Help-seeking: A review of the literature. *American Journal of Community Psychology, 6,* 413-424.

Hein, K. (1993). "Getting real" about HIV in adolescents. *American Journal of Public Health, 83*(4),492-494.

Hill, R. (1971). *Strengths of black families.* New York: Everson Hall Publishers.

Israel, B. (1985). Social networks and social support: Implications for natural helper and community level interventions. *Health Education Quarterly, 12* (1), 65-80.

Kral, A., Molnar, B., Booth, R., and Watters, J. (1997). Prevalence of sexual risk behaviour and substance use among runaway and homeless adolescents in San Francisco, Denver and New York City. *International Journal of STD & AIDS, 8,* 109-117.

Le Roux, J. (1996). Street children in South Africa: Findings from interviews on the background of street children in Pretoria, South Africa. *Adolescence, 31* (122), 423-431.

McAdoo, H. (Ed.) (1981). *Black families.* Beverly Hills, CA: Sage Publications.

Morse, E., Simon, P., and Burchfiel, K. (1999). Social environment and male sex work in the United States. In Aggleton, P. (Ed.). *Men who sell sex: International perspectives on male prostitution and HIV/AIDS.* Philadelphia, PA: Temple University Press.

Newman, P. (1999). Coming out positive? HIV prevention for gay, lesbian, and bisexual youths. In Shernoff, M. (Ed.). *AIDS and mental health practice: Clinical and policy issues.* New York: The Haworth Press, Inc.

Pennbridge, J., Yates, G., David, T. et al. (1990). Runaway and homeless youth in Los Angeles County, California. *Journal of Adolescent Health Care, 11,* 159-165.

Perry, C. and Sieving, R. (1991). *Peer involvement in global AIDS prevention among adolescents.* Geneva, Switzerland: Global Programme on AIDS World Health Organization.

Pfeffer, R. (1997). *Surviving the streets: Girls living on their own.* New York & London: Garland Publishing, Inc.

Raffaelli, M. (1997). The family situation of street youth in Latin America: A cross-national review. *International Social Work, 40,* 89-100.

Richter, L. (1991). Street children in South Africa. *Child Care Worker, 9,* 5-7.

Riordan, R. (1992). Marginalised youth and unemployment. In Everatt, D. and Sisulu, E. (Eds.). *Black youth in crisis: Facing the future.* Braamfontein: Raven Press.

Rotheram-Borus, M., Feldman, J., Rosario, M. et al. (1994). Preventing HIV among runaways: Victims and victimization. In DiClemente, R. (Ed.). *Preventing AIDS: Theories and methods of behavioral interventions* (175-188). New York: Plenum.

Rotheram-Borus, M., O'Keefe, Z., Kracker, R. & Foo, H. (2000). Prevention of HIV among adolescents. *Prevention Science, 1,* 15-30.

Rotheram-Borus, M., Lee, M., Murphy, D. et al. (2001). Efficacy of a preventive intervention for youths living with HIV. *American Journal of Public Health, 91* (3), 400-407.

Scharff, W., Powell, M., and Thomas, E. (1986). Strollers-Street children of Cape Town. In Burman, S. and Reynolds, P. (Eds.). *Growing up in a divided society: The contexts of childhood in South Africa.* Johannesburg: Raven Press.

See, L. (1986). *Tensions and tangles between Afro Americans and Southeast Asian refugees.* Atlanta, GA: Wright Publishing Company, Inc.

Smit, G. and Liebenberg, L. (2000). The inner-city street child: A profile of the dilemma and some guidelines. *Social Work/Maatskaplike Werk, 36* (1), 25-34.

Snell, C. (1995). *Young men in the street: Help-seeking behavior of young male prostitutes.* Westport, CT: Praeger Publishers.

Sondheimer, D. (1992). HIV infection and disease among homeless adolescents. In DiClemente, R. (Ed.). *Adolescents and AIDS: A generation in jeopardy.* Newbury Park, CA: Sage Publications.

Sorensen, W., Lopez, L., and Anderson, P. (2001). Latino AIDS immigrants in the Western Gulf States: A different population and the need for innovative prevention strategies. *Journal of Health and Social Policy, 13* (1), 1-19.

Sugerman, S., Hergenroeder, A., Chacko, M., and Parcel, G. (1991). AIDS and adolescents: Knowledge, attitudes and behaviors of runaway and homeless youths. *American Journal of Diseases in Children, 145,* 431-436.

Swart-Kruger, J. and Richter, L. (1997). AIDS-related knowledge, attitudes and behaviour among South African street youth: Reflections on power, sexuality and the autonomous self. *Social Science Medicine, 45* (6), 957-966.

Thom, D. (1991). Adolescence. In Louw, D. (Ed.). *Human development.* Pretoria: HAUM Tertiary.

Vaux, A., Riedel, S., and Stewart, D. (1987). Modes of social support: The social support behaviors (SS-B) scale. *American Journal of Community Psychology, 15* (2), 209-237.

Walters, A. (1999). HIV prevention in street youth. *Journal of Adolescent Health, 25* (3), 187-198.

Arthritis and the Role of the Physician in Nonmalignant Pain and Disability

Carlton E. Miller, MD, FACR

SUMMARY. Most adults will experience at least one episode of low back pain. It is the second most common symptom that prompts visits to the doctor's office. Back pain is subjective and often presents with few objective findings on a physical exam. It remains a diagnostic and therapeutic challenge to many practitioners. Psychosocial and economic issues, such as litigation, workers' compensation claims and depression may have an impact on the management and treatment outcomes (*Helfgott, MD, Simon M., 2001*). Workers' compensation programs have a mandate to compensate only those who deserve compensation. Therefore, disability rating exists to sort out those who cannot work from those who will not work (*Sullivan, MD, 1992*). When treating chronic nonmalignant pain the physician should make a decision to either function as the patient's advocate or the rater of the patient's limitations. This will increase the likelihood of a healthy patient-physician relationship during what may be a very vulnerable and stressful period. It is very important to obtain sound acceptable documentation of the diseased patient's limitations by choosing the proper cost effective diagnostic studies, which are appropriate for each individual case. This will result in establishing

---

Carlton E. Miller is a Fellow of American College of Rheumatology, and affiliated with the Department of Internal Medicine, Southside Regional Medical Center, Petersburg, VA 23803. Dr. Miller is Clinical Assistant Professor of Medicine, Division of Rheumatology, Health Science Center, University of Virginia, Charlottesville, VA 22902.

[Haworth co-indexing entry note]: "Arthritis and the Role of the Physician in Nonmalignant Pain and Disability." Miller, Carlton E. Co-published simultaneously in *Journal of Health & Social Policy* (The Haworth Press, Inc.) Vol. 16, No. 1/2, 2002, pp. 33-42; and: *Disability and the Black Community* (ed: Sheila D. Miller) The Haworth Press, Inc., 2002, pp. 33-42. Single or multiple copies of this article are available for a fee from The Haworth Document Delivery Service [1-800-HAWORTH, 9:00 a.m. - 5:00 p.m. (EST). E-mail address: docdelivery@haworthpressc.com].

10.1300/J045v16n01_04

an accurate and correct diagnosis. This process should lead to offering the patient treatment options designed to achieve pain reduction and improvement of his/her activity of daily living. *[Article copies available for a fee from The Haworth Document Delivery Service: 1-800-HAWORTH. E-mail address: <docdelivery@haworthpress.com> Website: <http://www.HaworthPress.com> © 2002 by The Haworth Press, Inc. All rights reserved.]*

KEYWORDS. Rating, physician, treating physician, impairments

DISABILITY RATINGS

Low back pain is an uncomfortable sensation in the lumbar and buttock regions originating from neurons near or around the spinal canal that are injured or irritated by one or more pathologic processes. Pain is subjective and difficult to compare either qualitatively or quantitatively from person to person (*Casey, MD, 2001*).

Disability ratings are necessary for the Department of Labor and Industries (L & I) to effect claim closure and to end their obligation for wage replacement and health care cost. Having a treating physician hired specifically for the purpose to perform these evaluations offered a clear advantage to L & I in efficiency and cost savings when compared to a "panel of examiners" (*Sullivan, MD, 1992*). Low back pain is the most common cause of work-related disability in people under 45 years of age and the most expensive cause of work-related disability, in terms of workers' compensation and medical expenses (*Deyo, MD, 2001; Deyo, MD, 1987*). It is the second leading cause of all physician visits and the most frequent complaint among patients when they first visit a rheumatologist (*Deyo, MD, 1987*). About two thirds of adults suffer from low back pain at some time (*Deyo, MD, 2001*). The treating physicians should not do ratings, because the roles of the treating and rating physician are not compatible in the case of chronic pain. In addition, the measurement of disability due to pain through physician ratings is probably invalid (*Sullivan, MD, 1992*). For these reasons we will further discuss chronic nonmalignant pain and the issues that occur when disability determination is sought.

OSTEOARTHRITIS AND DISABILITY

Osteoarthritis is the most common form of arthritis that affects synovial joints. Most people who are 65 years or older will have some radiographic or pathological findings, which are related to osteoarthritis. The prevalence of osteoarthritis increases steeply with age. This condition initially was expected to occur with aging (*Badley PhD, 1995; Manek, MD, 2001*). Estimates reveal that 15 percent of Americans have some type of arthritis (mainly osteoarthritis), and of these, 15% have limitation of activities (*Biundo, Jr., MD, 2001*). Risk factors of low back pain include heavy lifting and twisting, bodily vibration, obesity, and poor muscle conditioning. Low back pain is also common even in people without these risk factors (*Deyo, MD, 2001*). Approximately 2% to 8% of patients develop chronic disabling pain. Seventy-five percent of all compensation payments in the United States go to patients with low back pain (*Helfgott, MD, Simon, M., 2001*). Treatment options were limited. The most common complaints by patients with this disorder were joint pain and decreased joint function (*Manek, MD, 2001*). The patients' individual values and intensity of their belief in hopes, fears and moods all motivate and crucially shape their capacity to function in the face of pain (*Sullivan, MD, 1992*). These symptoms are aggravated with weight bearing, and are improved with rest. Some patients developed joint pain, which gradually increases in frequency and duration until the pain is constant (*Manek, MD, 2001*). The most common example of chronic nonmalignant pain is low back pain (*Sullivan, MD, 1992*). Lower back pain affects men and women equally, with most people who reach the age of 60 years old experiencing episodes of back pain (*Deyo, MD, 2001; Hadler, MD, 2001*). Lower back pain is the most common cause of disability in the working years and one of the most expensive health care problems in the industrialized world (*Sullivan, MD, 1992*). Many people never seek medical advice from a physician concerning their back pain until it becomes unbearable or persistent. Once their back pain begins to affect their activity of daily living, then the patients are willing to agree to allow investigative tests in order to establish a diagnosis. Low back pain is now the second most common reason a patient visits a primary care physician office (*Deyo, MD, 1987, Hadler, MD, 2001*). The vast majority of back pain is self-limited; resolution generally occurs without surgery or often any formal medical intervention. In a small but financially significant group of patients, back pain persists despite conservative and/or surgical treatment (*Sullivan, MD, 1992*). The pursuit of inpatient or outpatient medical services not only results in high medical cost, but it also results in increased time from work, which is an indirect medical cost (*Hadler, MD, 2001*). A study conducted by Deyo and Tsui-Wu showed a trend of more frequent hospitalizations among those patients with less education (*Deyo, MD, 1987*). The patient in the African-American community continues to need and rely on the family as the major source of support and help. The family continues, especially today, to provide the comfort, understanding, and support needed to offset stress, strain, tensions, apprehensions, and anxieties (*Miller, DSW, 1993*). In addition to the high cost of treating these disorders, missed workdays also result in loss of income, which may result in anxiety and the inability to function at home (*Hadler, MD, 2001*).

WORKMAN'S COMPENSATION

All fifty (50) states have provided a system of workers' compensation, since 1949. Workers' compensation programs have a mandate to compensate only those who deserve compensation. Disability rating exists to sort out those who cannot work from those who will not work (*Sullivan, MD, 1992*). The rate of arthritis-associated disability is projected to increase in all the new world countries (*Badley, PhD, 1995*). Workman's compensation needs to know how an injury specifically affects the patient's ability to work. No longer must an employee prove why he was injured, but he must still prove that he became injured on the job, and that this injury produces an inability to work so that he would qualify for wage replacement. Society has turned to physicians to help to sort out compensable from non-compensable disability due to injury (*Sullivan, 1992*). Three prominent goals or outcomes that are possible for the clinical encounter with the injured worker with chronic pain are relief of suffering, return to work, and closure of the case for compensation purposes. The physician who is in the role of treating or rating, does not prioritize these goals in the same way (*Sullivan, MD, 1992*). Prolonged back pain may be associated with the failure of previous treatment, depression, and somatization. Substance abuse, job dissatisfaction, pursuit of disability compensation, and involvement in litigation may also be associated with persistent unexplained symptoms (*Deyo, MD, 2001*). The availability of additional support systems and degree of involvement in the community may result in the African-American disabled person, at times, not engaging or participating in traditional treatment (*Miller, DSW, 1993*). The treating physicians are primarily interested in relief of suffering through treatment of the underlying disease.

Case closure in this setting relates to return to work because of the relief of suffering. On the other hand, ratings are conducted in inverse relationship to this priority. Case closure is the primary goal because rating exists for determining liability. The role of a rater return to work promotes case closure and relief of suffering is of interest because it allows return to work (*Sullivan, MD, 1992*). This process is not meant to portray the workers' compensation system as heartless. It is only to emphasize that it is a system to redress work injury as the reason that limits return to work. It is not a system of medical care, or medical insurance. When the cause and cure of disability are clear, as in the case with most workplace injuries, these systems blend reasonably well. When the cause and cure are difficult to define, as in the case of disability related to chronic pain, there is the potential for a complicated and confrontational inter-action (*Sullivan, MD, 1992*).

PHYSICIANS' ROLE IN DISABILITY

There are similarities in the line of questioning used by the rating and treat-ing physician in obtaining diagnostic information from patients who are in the disability process. According to the AMA Guides to the Evaluation of Perma-nent Impairment, the first key to effective and reliable evaluation of a patient's impairment is to review the office and hospital records since the onset of the medical condition (*Sullivan, 1992*). The precise pathoanatomical diagnosis is difficult to localize and isolate in 85% of patients with low back pain. Common problems seen in lower back pain include disk herniation and spinal stenois, which is when the disk material or bony osteophytes cause narrowing of the central spinal canal area (*Deyo, MD, 2001*). Patients tend to reveal information more readily to their treating physician than to a physician whom they see solely for disability rating. When a physician accepts the responsibility of both roles, this is the first area where trouble begins. The physician as rater is not only borrowing knowledge obtained through his role as treating physician, but he is borrowing the patient's trust as well. Encounters between physician and patient for the purposes of treating and rating disability create fundamentally different relationships. Some physicians believe the doctor-patient relation-ship can be preserved by simple honesty of the physician shifting allegiance. The patient can adjust by temporarily treating the physician as an adversary rather than an advocate. It may be possible for patients to decrease their level of trust within this relationship, but it is difficult to "upgrade" their trust again. Physicians are told they are rating impairment, yet they are asked to comment on disability. When the purpose for establishing the medical diagnosis is to se-lect an effective treatment for the patient's pain, the physician is acting as an agent for the patient (*Sullivan, 1992*). Nonspecific terms, such as strain, sprain, or degenerative processes, are commonly used. These terms do not have ana-tomically or histologically bases, and patients given these diagnoses may be said to have idiopathic low back pain. In recent years, magnetic resonance im-aging (MRI) has come to be widely used to document objective findings that support the claims of the patients (*Deyo, MD, 2001*). When the purpose of de-termining the diagnosis is to rate the patient's disability, then the physician acts as an agent for the state. The purpose for the former encounter is to reduce suffering; the purpose of the latter encounter is to assign compensation as man-dated by law or regulation. If two different physicians perform this task, there is little chance for confusion about the nature of the relationship between the physician and the patient (*Sullivan, 1992*). Patients may be less candid if they sense that their physician is doing some "police work" for the institution. A more awkward situation occurs when the patient is not aware that the physician has switched allegiance (*Sullivan, MD, 1992*). If patients perceive any confusion of the role of their physician, then not only is candor hindered, but also the trust in the integrity in their physician compromised (*Sullivan, MD, 1992*).

DISABILITY RATING

Disability rating is designed to determine who deserves compensation. This evaluation is done whenever the injured worker cannot or will not perform a particular function, which is associated with their job (*Sullivan, MD, 1992*). Return to work after an episode of low back pain is influenced by clinical, social, and economic factors. Low back pain is rarely permanently disabling (*Deyo, MD, 2001*). The distinction between cannot and will not is especially difficult in patients suffering from chronic pain. Patients with chronic pain have not lost function per se, as in paresis, but they have lost comfortable function (*Sullivan, MD, 1992*). Recovery from nonspecific low back pain is generally rapid. In one study, 90% of patients seen within three days of onset recovered within two weeks (*Deyo, MD, 2001*). Pain blurs the difference between cannot and will not by making function difficult, but not impossible.

The strategy for disability ratings advocated by the World Health Organization (WHO) and the AMA for separating compensable and non-compensable loss of function relies on the distinction between impairment and disability. The WHO defines impairment as "any loss or abnormality of psychological, physiological, or anatomical structure or function." Disability is defined as a disadvantage for a given individual (resulting from an impairment or functional limitation) that limits or prevents fulfillment of a role that is normal for that individual related to age, sex, social and cultural factors. Impairment is the absolute loss of function, while disability is the inability to meet the expectations of a certain role (*Biundo, Jr., MD, 2001; Sullivan, MD, 1992*).

An important feature to note concerning impairment is that it is not fixed and static following an injury. Rehabilitation efforts change impairments whether they originate with a stroke, knee surgery, or a back injury at work (*Sullivan, MD, 1992*). A rehabilitation program can ameliorate impairment and resulting disability caused by rheumatic diseases even when the disease remains active (*Biundo, Jr., MD, 2001*). Impairment is an anatomic or functional abnormality or loss of function after achieving maximal medical rehabilitation, determined by the patient's values, goals, and motivations. Patient value determines which impairments are disabling. The patient's effort is a crucial element in rehabilitative care, and determining the level of impairment ultimately produced by the injury (*Sullivan, MD, 1992*).

TREATMENT STRATEGIES

There are many pain reduction strategies offered to patients as alternatives to medications. Relaxation, distraction, and, most importantly, increased levels of exercise are utilized with the aim of putting the patients themselves back in control of their pain and their lives (*Sullivan, MD, 1992*). Most patients want a quick fix and a promise that their back pain will not return (*Hadler, MD, 2001*). Conventional traction, facet-joint injections, and transcutaneous electrical nerve stimulation appear ineffective or minimally effective in randomized trials. Infrequently studies show very little support for acupuncture and the usefulness of massage (*Deyo, MD, 2001*). Strategies used for the palliation of acute pain, such as narcotics and sedatives, are also often counterproductive when used to treat chronic pain caused by nonmalignant disorders. Rather than promoting healing, these drugs can produce lethargy, apathy, physical dependence, and depression (*Sullivan, MD, 1992*). Counseling continues to be identified as extremely helpful and a major strength to the disabled patient and his/her family. The lack of available appropriate services and resources directly affects the counseling process and hinders the coping skills of both patients and family. Disabled African-American patients continue to function with whatever support the family, their community and friends can provide (Miller, DSW, 1993).

The goals of management of osteoarthritis were outlined in the 1995 American College of Rheumatology (ACR) guidelines, which are: to control pain, maintain or improve joint mobility, minimize disability and educate patients and their families about their disease and its treatments (*Manek, MD, 2001*). Therapeutic success depends in many ways on trust between the physician and patient, especially in a rehabilitation setting, in which the patients values and motivation play such a central role (*Sullivan, MD, 1992*).

Clinical studies of low back pain vary widely in the type of outcomes used to assess the success of therapies. A standard set of outcome measures would make it easier to compare the magnitude of treatment effects across studies. The Roland Morris Disability Questionnaire (RDQ) and the Oswestry Disability Index (ODI) are examples of the two most commonly used specific measures of function in lower back pain (*Bombardies, MD, 2001*). The management of osteoarthritis is subdivided into non-medical or non-pharmacological therapy and drug or pharmacological treatments. Surgical treatments include:

diskectomy, laminectomy, nerve blocks, joint lavage, osteotomy and total joint arthroplasty. Surgery is offered to the patient who has failed medical management and when functional disability has began to affect that patient's quality of life (*Deyo, MD, 2001; Manek, MD, 2001*). For example, diskectomy produced better pain relief than non-surgical treatment over a period of four years but it is unclear whether there is any advantage after 10 years (*Deyo, MD, 2001*).

Currently the standard treatment for lower back pain is the conservative approach, which includes bed rest for no more than one or two days, nonsteroidal anti-inflammatory drugs (NSAIDs) and exercise. Bed rest should be brief and patients should return to their normal activities as soon as possible (*Hadler, MD, 2001*). Non-pharmacologic modalities are the cornerstone of management of osteoarthritis of the hip and of the knee. There is an association between obesity and osteoarthritis. It is most pronounced in overweight postmenopausal women. The 1995 ACR guidelines recommended that patients who are obese and have osteoarthritis of the hip or knee should lose weight (*Manek, MD, 2001*). The relationship between loss of body fat and improvement in symptoms of osteoarthritis of the knee exist (*ACR Subcommittee on OA Guidelines, 2000 Update; Manek, MD, 2001*). Manipulation is very useful when a patient presents with acute lower back pain, such that the onset of symptoms does not exceed one to three months in duration. Manipulation offered to patients who have recent onset of lower back pain but not to a patient who has radicular symptoms is acceptable. Radicular symptoms would suggest that the spinal cord or nerve roots are involved. The patient should be re-evaluated and manipulative therapy stopped if functional or symptomatic improvement has not been achieved. The diagnosis of mechanical back pain or chronic regional back pain can be made only after all serious illnesses and disorders have been ruled out (*Hadler, MD, 2001*). Bed rest is not recommended for the treatment of low back pain or sciatica, and a rapid return to normal activities is usually the best course (*Deyo, MD, 2001*). Special tests are reserved for patients who have diseases that are more specific. Most patients who have mechanical back pain recover or their symptoms resolve with conservative treatments (*Hadler, MD, 2001*).

Osteopathic manipulation has been accepted in the medical community as an appropriate treatment for acute low back pain. There are about 42,000 licensed osteopathic physicians and 55,000 licensed chiropractors in this country. Osteopathic doctors account for about 5% of the entire physician population in the United States of America. They provide holistic care with emphasis on structure and function. Not all osteopathic physicians practice manipulation as part of their medical care (*Hadler, MD, 2001*).

Physical therapists are licensed health care professionals who assess changes in the strength, endurance, coordination, and mobility of the soft tissue or joints. They have a wide variety of methods and modalities to use to treat this category of patients. In addition to manual therapy, they utilize active and passive exercise and movements, self-care education, and physical agents (thermal treatments, traction and water) (*Hadler, MD, 2001*). Exercise may be the most effective and inexpensive physical intervention available for reducing joint pain and impairment in patients with osteoarthritis. Therapeutic exercises fall in three (3) categories, which are range of motion and flexibility, muscle conditioning, and aerobic cardiovascular exercises. The most current exercise research has been focused in osteoarthritis of the hip and the knee, because they account for most of the disabling osteoarthritis diagnoses. Quadriceps weakness is common among patients with knee osteoarthritis. Isometric exercises to strengthen the quadriceps muscles are beneficial (*Manek, MD, 2001*). Clinical evidence that demonstrates that physical therapy or massage therapy for lower back pain is effective is limited. It is important to realize that if a patient has been receiving manual therapies without objective evidence of improvement after three to four weeks of care, then the method of treatment should be discontinued and the patient reassessed (*Hadler, MD, 2001*). Referral to a multidisciplinary pain center may be appropriate for some patients with chronic low back pain. Such centers typically combine cognitive-behavioral therapy, patient education, supervised exercise, selective nerve blocks and other strategies to restore functioning (*Deyo, MD, 2001*).

CONCLUSION

The physician should select the role that provides the best service for their patient who has chronic pain, work injury and disability issues. This review has illustrated that conflicts are more likely to occur between patients and their doctor when their physician assumes the dual role of treating and rating. Having your personal physician maintain the position of patient advocate and having information forwarded to a separate rating physician may preserve the doctor patient relationship. This becomes important when evaluating and treating chronic nonmalignant pain in relationship to return to work issues. Some patients may still elect to request their physician to complete brief forms to comment on their level of impairment, but a discussion concerning roles should occur if disability-related determination issues arise.

Objective findings are encouraged when clarifying the extent of impairments and disability in order to achieve closure for return to work issues and closure of impairment and disability episodes. Anatomical studies and functional assessment documentation are necessary to retain focus on the overall goals needed to approach the unification of criteria accepted by Workman's Compensation, the patients' impairment and their belief of their disability for closure of return-to-work issues.

REFERENCES

American College of Rheumatology Subcommittee on Osteoarthritis Guidelines. Recommendations for the Medical Management of Osteoarthritis of the Hip and Knee: 2000 Update, *Arthritis and Rheumatism, 2000;* Vol 43, P. 1905-1915.

Badley, PhD, Elizabeth M., Crotty, MD, Maria, An International Comparison of the Estimated Effect of the Aging of the Population on the Major Cause of Disablement, Musculoskeletal Disorders, *The Journal of Rheumatology,* Vol 22: No 10 (April 1995), P.1934-1940.

Biundo, Jr., MD, Joseph J., Rush, MD, Perry J., Rehabilitation of Patients with Rheumatic Diseases, *Kelley's Textbook of Rheumatology,* 6th ed, 2001, P. 763-775.

Bombardier, MD, FRCP, Claire, Hayden, BSc, DC, Jill, Beaton BScOT, MSc, PhD, Minimal Clinically Important Difference, Low Back Pain: Outcome Measures, *The Journal of Rheumatology,* 2001, Vol 28, No 2, P. 431-438.

Casey, MD, Patrick, Weinstein, MD, James N., Low Back Pain, *Kelley's Textbook of Rheumatology,* 6th ed, 2001, P. 509-523.

Deyo, MD, MPH, Richard A., Tsui-Wu, Yuh-Jane, MS, Functional Disability due to Back Pain, *Arthritis and Rheumatism,* Vol. 30, No. 11 (November 1987), P. 1247-1253.

Deyo, MD, MPH, Richard A., Weinstein, DO, James N. *New England Journal of Medicine,* Vol. 344, No. 5, February 1, 2001, P. 363-370.

Hadler, MD, Nortin, M., Pearson, DO, Jeffrey K., Shekelle, MD, PhD. Manual Therapy for Low Back Pain. *Patient Care.* May 30, 2001; P. 12-23.

Helfgott, MD, Simon M. Sensible Approach to Low Back Pain, *Bulletin on the Rheumatic Diseases,* Vol 50, No 3, P. 1-4, 2001.

Manek, MD, Nisha J., Medical Management of Osteoarthritis, *Mayo Clinic Proceedings.* May 2001, Vol 76, Number 5, P. 533-539.

Miller, DSW, Sheila D., Increasing the Adjustment Success of the Disabled African American. *Journal of Health & Social Policy,* Vol 5(2) P. 87-103. 1993.

Sullivan, MD, PhD, Mark D., Loeser, MD, John D., The Diagnosis of Disability Treating and Rating Disability in a Pain Clinic, *Archives of Internal Medicine.* September 1992. Vol 152, P. 1829-1835.

The Context of Religiosity, Social Support and Health Locus of Control: Implications for the Health-Related Quality of Life of African-American Hemodialysis Patients

Claudie J. Thomas, ABD, MSW

SUMMARY. Most African-Americans choose hemodialysis as a treatment regimen when diagnosed with renal failure modality. Some researchers suggest that African-American hemodialysis patients' health-related quality of life enables them to cope with and survive this type of difficult renal therapy better than other racial and ethnic groups. This article examines how the sociocultural and social psychological constructs of religiosity, social support and health locus of control, relate to the health-related quality of life for this population group. *[Article copies available for a fee from The Haworth Document Delivery Service: 1-800-HAWORTH. E-mail address: <docdelivery@haworthpress.com> Website: <http://www.HaworthPress. com> © 2002 by The Haworth Press, Inc. All rights reserved.]*

KEYWORDS. African-American, biopsychosocial, ecological framework, health locus of control, health-related quality of life, hemodialysis, holism,

Claudie J. Thomas is Adjunct Professor, Ethelyn R. Strong School of Social Work, Norfolk State University, Norfolk, VA.

[Haworth co-indexing entry note]: "The Context of Religiosity, Social Support and Health Locus of Control: Implications for the Health-Related Quality of Life of African-American Hemodialysis Patients." Thomas, Claudie J. Co-published simultaneously in *Journal of Health & Social Policy* (The Haworth Press, Inc.) Vol. 16, No. 1/2, 2002, pp. 43-54; and: *Disability and the Black Community* (ed: Sheila D. Miller) The Haworth Press, Inc., 2002, pp. 43-54. Single or multiple copies of this article are available for a fee from The Haworth Document Delivery Service [1-800-HAWORTH, 9:00 a.m. - 5:00 p.m. (EST). E-mail address: docdelivery@haworthpress.com].

religiosity, renal failure, social support, social systems theory, strengths perspective

INTRODUCTION

The health-related quality of life of African-American hemodialysis patients is an issue that needs more attention. The increased incidence of chronic diseases such as hypertension and diabetes has led to a proliferation of African-Americans who suffer renal (kidney) failure. The data show that renal failure in African-American communities is approximately three times the rate in the general population. Therefore, this increases the need for renal replacement therapy (Price & Owen, 1997).

Once confronted with renal failure, individuals have options regarding treatment modalities. Hemodialysis is one option for the treatment of end-stage renal disease. Approximately 90% of African-Americans choose hemodialysis as a treatment modality (Price & Owen, 1997). Even though African-Americans choose hemodialysis at a high rate, this treatment modality is often fraught with rigors and difficulties in attempting to maintain a positive outlook on life. These include physiological changes and psychosocial issues (Furr, 1998).

STATEMENT OF THE PROBLEM

With all the difficulties associated with hemodialysis, it has been suggested that African-Americans cope with and survive this process better than other racial and ethnic groups (Price & Owen, 1997). Among the explanations Price and Owen (1997) cite for this phenomenon are that African-Americans undergoing hemodialysis exhibit a greater satisfaction with life overall which results in an improved quality of life. These researchers consider African-American hemodialysis patients' health-related quality of life to be a factor in their ability to cope with the hardships of this particular type of renal therapy. However, they are at a loss to explain why African-Americans enjoy a relatively stable health-related quality of life. Consequently, Leggat, Swartz and Port (1997) suggest that sociocultural factors help to explain why African-Americans undergoing the hemodialysis treatment regimen maintain good health-related quality of life.

Sociocultural factors have not been used extensively to explain why African-American hemodialysis patients seem to exhibit good health-related quality of life. However, seminal research conducted by Hill (1971) and Stack (1974) posits that religion (Hill) and kinship networks (Hill & Stack) have helped African-Americans cope with various deleterious situations in this society. Additionally, Neighbors and Jackson (1996) suggest that for African-Americans, a deterministic outlook on life may be beneficial in attempting to cope with life's challenges.

Thus, a strong religious orientation, a well-defined social network alliance which provides support and an external direction relative to control of one's health may yield explanatory power for the health-related quality of life of African-American hemodialysis patients. Consequently, the problem can be stated as: what is the effect of religiosity, the impact of social support and the significance of health locus of control on the health-related quality of life of African-American hemodialysis patients?

PROBLEM SIGNIFICANCE

Although the incidence of renal failure for African-Americans is approximately three times that of the general population (Price & Owen, 1997), very few studies have focused specifically on the health-related quality of life of this population (Leggat et al., 1997). Studies that have examined race in relationship to hemodialysis or end-stage renal disease have used it mostly as a background or demographic variable (Holder, 1997).

Another area of significance is the sociocultural aspect of health-related quality of life of African-American hemodialysis patients. Holder (1997) and Leggat et al. (1997) postulate that cultural components of African-Americans on maintenance dialysis allow this population to face the demands imposed by their hemodialysis treatment regimen. Thus, these researchers assert that church involvement, extended family, community and organizational ties, along with prolonged experience with adversity, affect this population's health-related quality of life. However, they believe that further research and exploration of this phenomenon is warranted due to the paucity of existing research studies.

LITERATURE REVIEW

The few studies that have been conducted on African-American hemodialysis patients' health-related quality of life have basically compared African-Americans and whites (Leggat et al., 1997). Tell, Shumaker, Mittlemark et al. (1995) and Kutner and Devins (1998) found that African-American end-stage renal disease/hemodialysis patients enjoyed a higher health-related quality of life than white patients. However, these researchers could not fully explain the reasons for this phenomenon. They did surmise, however, that culture, life experiences and attitudes toward health might play a significant role in African-American hemodialysis and end-stage renal disease patients' health-related quality of life. Therefore, these researchers suggest that other investigators conduct more in-depth analyses to determine what factors, especially sociocultural components, such as religiosity and social support, contribute to African-American hemodialysis patients' health-related quality of life (Kutner & Devins, 1998; Tell et al., 1995).

A review of empirical studies of hemodialysis patients' health-related quality of life reveals that only a few studies include religiosity/spirituality as a component of their research (Mathews, 1998). Ferrans and Powers (1993) found that personal faith in God had the highest correlation (r = .50) of any other variables in relationship to life satisfaction for hemodialysis patients. Mathews (1998) cites a study by O'Brien (1982) in which the investigators found that 51% of end-stage renal disease patients attended religious services monthly and 20% attended some type of religious services weekly.

In regards to religiosity and African-Americans, the strong emphasis on religiosity by African-Americans and the role of the Black church in stabilizing and sustaining African-American communities was documented by Drake and Cayton (1945), Frazier (1974) and Woodson (1939) as cited in Taylor and Chatters (1991). Additionally, the Black church assumed many roles denied to African-Americans by the wider society. These included educational, philanthropic, civic, social and business functions (Boyd-Franklin & Bry, 2000). Additionally, other researchers, including Brown and Gary (1994) and Ellison and Taylor (1996), have concluded through their studies, that religiosity does have a positive impact on health for African-Americans.

For hemodialysis and end-stage renal disease patients, researchers have also found that social support has a significant impact on the health-related quality of life for this population. These researchers, including Elal and Krespi (1999) and Tell et al. (1995), found that various aspects of social support help hemodialysis and end-stage renal disease patients cope better with the treatment regimen.

Several empirical studies of social support and African-Americans by scholars such as Hill (1972), Manns (1997), Stack (1974), and Taylor, Hardison and Chatters (1996) lend credibility to the thesis that familial and non-familial relationships of African-Americans provide sustenance and support to African-Americans in need. Other studies also reveal that social support also influences health-promotive behavior among African-Americans (Belgrave & Lewis, 1994; Neighbors & Jackson, 1984).

In reference to locus of control, Rotter developed this construct through a series of studies on perceived control (Skinner, 1995). The locus of control construct can also be applied to health behavior and health belief. For hemodialysis/end-stage renal disease patients, however, studies on dietary/fluid adherence and health locus of control have yielded inconsistent and inconclusive results (Furr, 1998).

There are a couple of omissions in the literature relative to African-American hemodialysis patients. First, is the use of non-comparative studies of African-American hemodialysis patients (Leggatt et al., 1997). Very few studies specifically focus on African-Americans in the end-stage renal disease population. Instead, most of the studies compare African-Americans and whites when addressing issues of health-related quality of life in the end-stage renal disease/hemodialysis population (Leggatt et al., 1997).

Secondly, the use of sociocultural propositions to help explain health-related quality of life in the African-American hemodialyis/end-stage renal disease population is slight. Thus, constructs such as the extended kinship network and the importance of religion in many African-American communities have not been examined fully. Hence, sociocultural factors related to health-related quality of life, in addition to the somatic influences, should be more fully investigated (Holder, 1997; Leggatt et al., 1997). In order to accomplish this, the manner in which health-related quality of life is conceptualized should be broadened to include psychosocial parameters (Furr, 1998). Consequently, the theoretical underpinnings of health-related quality of life, religiosity, social support and health locus of control will be examined.

CONCEPTUAL FOUNDATIONS
OF HEALTH-RELATED QUALITY OF LIFE

Health-related quality of life is a multidimensional construct that embodies spiritual, psychological, physical, social and community belonging. The construct combines the broad definition of health with a sense of general well-being and life satisfaction. Hence, the construct is of a biopsychosocial nature which can best be understood through the interrelated concepts of social systems theory, the ecological framework, the strengths perspective and holistic concepts (Raeburn & Rootman, 1996).

Social systems theory focuses on the interaction, mutuality and reciprocity between humans (Kirst-Ashman & Hull, 1999). The ecological perspective centers on reciprocity, or how system components influence each other, and adaptation, the ability of individuals to transform or reshape themselves or their environments in order to maintain balance and equilibrium (Germain & Bloom, 1999). The guiding precepts of the strengths perspective are a belief in the worth and dignity of each individual and the notion of resilience, or the ability of individuals to recover and recuperate from devastating and traumatic events (Saleeby, 1996). Holism focuses on the balance and interconnectedness among the physical, social, psychological and spiritual entities. Consequently, the main principle in holism is wholeness, or the unity and oneness of mind, body and spirit (Patterson, 1998).

Any conceptual framework that has relevance to African-Americans' health-related quality of life must take into account the strength, resiliency and cultural patterns of this population (Airhihenbuwa, 1995). Whereas the strengths perspective, social systems theory, the ecological perspective and holism are all underlying concepts of health-related quality of life (Raeburn & Rootman, 1996), they are also relevant to health issues and other concerns in African-American communities (Littlejohn-Blake and Darling, 1993; Miller, 1993).

Hill's landmark study that outlines the strengths of African-American families is a prime example of how the strengths perspective can be relevant to African-American health issues (Miller, 1993). Boyd-Franklin and Bry's (2000) Multisystems framework is an example of social systems theory being applied to the study of African-American family life. Miller (1993) applies the concept of adaptation from the ecological perspective to the adjustment process of African-Americans with chronic illnesses and disabilities. Finally, holism is relevant to the study of African-American family life because it allows scholars and researchers to assess this population in a comprehensive manner (Taylor, Jackson & Chatters, 1997). In summary, the strengths perspective, social systems theory, ecological perspective and holism are conceptual cornerstones in African-American family studies (Littlejohn-Blake & Darling, 1993).

RELIGIOSITY AND HEALTH

The concept of religion centers on a set of presuppositions, experiences, customs and obligations used by groups to create philosophical notions of life. Thus, religion can be the search for the significance and sacredness of life, whereas religiosity is the individual trait possessed by the community of like believers (Levin & Schiller, 1987). Consequently, a major question confronting sociomedical researchers is how religiosity impacts health. One possible explanation is the epidemiological stage of salutogenesis in the pathogenesis model (Levin, 1996). With salutogenesis (Antonovsky, 1987) as cited in Levin (1996), protective factors can preclude pathogens from causing disease while simultaneously promoting health and well-being. Thus, religiosity may affect health through a protective mechanism that makes pathogenic symptomology difficult. Therefore, certain aspects of religiosity such as religious fervor, fellowship, prayer, faith and obedience may lead to protective factors for disease. These protective factors can include adherence to healthy diets, complementary support from fellow worshipers, an enhanced emotional state and a heightened holistic energy field (Levin, 1996).

SOCIAL SUPPORT AND HEALTH

In the 1970s, there was an exponential increase in the number of evidentiary studies that focused on social relationships and health, however there was less unanimity regarding the conceptualization of the construct (Bowling, 1997). Cohen and Syme (1985) simply define social support as "resources provided by other people" (p. 4). However, House's (1981) multidimensional conceptualization, as cited in Bowling (1997), focuses on four distinct functions of social support. These include emotional attention, instrumental assistance, information and appraisal.

Social support can also influence health directly (main effect) or indirectly (buffering) effect. In the main effect model, social support augments health regardless of the stress level. Thus, the aid provided by the network is consistent, constant and routine. With the buffering hypothesis, however, support offers individuals a protective shield only after a stressful event has occurred, such as a traumatic health crisis. Thus, the buffering hypothesis is a means of helping individuals cope with stressful health events (Lewis, Rook & Schwarzer, 1994).

Another social support conceptual dilemma relates to whether or not the social network should be defined according to structure or function. Structural characteristics generally refer to the network size and the degree of interaction among its members. The functional aspect of social support, however, pertains to a rendering of what the network actually provides. Thus, social support researchers who are concerned with functional characteristics would be interested in knowing whether the network provided emotional, information, instrumental or appraisal support. Furthermore, an individual's perception of available resources and the manner in which the resources are delivered also determine functional support (Bowling, 1997; Cohen & Syme, 1985).

LOCUS OF CONTROL AND HEALTH

Locus of control is a major construct under the larger theoretical heading of perceived control and was derived from Rotter's (1954) social learning theory (Skinner, 1995). Wallston, Wallston, Kaplan and Maides (1976) appropriated the construct specifically for health behaviors. In this context, individuals who believe that they have a degree of control over their health outcomes are more internally-oriented. Conversely, individuals who believe that luck, chance, fate or powerful others facilitate their health outcomes are more externally directed. Thus, according to this theory, those who are more internally-oriented are also more likely to be more proactive regarding their health behaviors (Reich, Erdal & Zautra, 1997).

Locus of Control and African-Americans

Neighbors and Jackson (1996) argue that many of the locus of control studies that negatively conclude that African-Americans possess an external, deterministic control orientation in comparison with whites are flawed. These researchers contend that many mental health theorists and researchers are much too concerned with the characteristics of the locus of control construct itself and are therefore oblivious to the differences by which the construct operates for African-Americans. For example, Neighbors and Jackson (1996) do not view an external orientation as entirely negative. They aver that the external orientation's system-blame focus has protective and coping functions in that it makes allowances for the realistic consequences of racism, oppression and discrimination. Consequently, the externality's system-blame characteristic can diffuse self-blame tendencies associated with internality that can be destructive to the individual psyche. Therefore, comparative analyses must be used judiciously, if at all, so that an entire population will not be denigrated based on this construct (1996).

IMPLICATIONS FOR SOCIAL WORK PRACTICE

During the past two decades this country has experienced rapid technological growth, especially in the medical sciences. Thus, medical science can now create life (to a certain point), sustain life, and prolong the end of life. However, one must ask whether this high technological medicine has brought sufficient improvement to the quality of the individual's life. These innovations can certainly sustain the physical body; however, the other components such as the social, emotional and spiritual must be actively engaged in life-affirming activities in order to enjoy good health-related quality of life (McGee & Bradley, 1994). Therefore, renal social workers should be extremely cognizant of the *quality* of those individuals' lives who undergo hemodialysis treatment for end-stage renal disease (Furr, 1998).

The social work profession's emphasis on holism, or the perspective that the individual is an aggregate of systems that work together (Skidmore et al., 1997), intersects with high technological medicine's limited accent on, mostly, the individual's physical being (McGee & Bradley, 1994). Whether medicine's ability to prolong life relates to renal failure, cancer, HIV/AIDS, heart disease or other maladies, social workers must be able to "treat" the whole person. This entails the physical, emotional, social and, increasingly, the spiritual aspect of the individual's being. Thus, social workers must develop a greater understanding of the complexities of holistic treatment as it relates to a comprehensive healing process, i.e., a rejuvenation of the individual's physical, emotional, social and spiritual selves (Harper, 1990).

The nexus of technological innovation in medicine with sociocultural components of the African-American hemodialysis patient population has additional implications for nephrology (renal) social workers. Although technological advances help prolong lives, sociocultural and social psychological elements add depth to the quality of those lives. Therefore, it is vitally important that nephrology social workers be enlightened regarding cultural adaptations to health and wellness, especially as they relate to African-American hemodialysis patients. Consequently, renal social workers, especially those not of color, must increase their awareness and sensitivity to African-American cultural attributes (Washington, 1999).

Also those social workers engaged in policy development must insure that the profession's stance on health-related quality of life is incorporated into the appropriation of quality of care and quality of life guidelines for the renal community. Thus, renal social workers involved in quality of care and quality of life policy initiatives must insure that clinical indicators are broadened to also measure how the emotional, social and spiritual elements contribute to an enhanced quality of life (Bradley & McGee, 1994). Additionally, if sound, rigorous research is conducted on the health-related quality of life of hemodialysis patients, social work researchers may be able to persuade health care planners to view quality of life in a more holistic manner (Furr, 1998; Washington, 1999).

In conclusion, sociocultural and social psychological constructs can have a significant impact on health-related quality of life (Raeburn & Rootman, 1996). Thus, for African-American hemodialysis patients, these sociocultural and social psychological constructs may be even more important in addressing health-related quality of life. Hopefully, more research studies will be undertaken to address these issues for this population (Leggat et al., 1997).

REFERENCES

Airhihenbuwa, C. O. (1995). *Health and culture: Beyond the western paradigm.* Thousand Oaks, CA: Sage Publications.
Belgrave, F. & Lewis, D. (1994). The role of social support in compliance and other health behaviors for African-Americans with chronic illness. *Journal of Health Social Policy, 5 (3-4)*, 55-68.

Bowling, A. (1997). *Measuring health: A review pf quality of life measurement scales. Second edition.* Buckingham, England: Open University Press.

Boyd-Franklin, N. & Bry, B. H. (2000). *Reaching out in family therapy: Home-based, school and community interventions.* New York: The Guilford Press.

Bradley, C. & McGee, H. (1994). Improving quality of life in renal failure: Ways forward. In McGee, H. & Bradley, C. (Eds). *Quality of life following renal failure.* Switzerland: Harwood Academic.

Brown, D. & Gary, L. (1994). Religious involvement and health status among African-American males. *Journal of the National Medical Association, 86 (11),* 824-831.

Cohen. S. & Syme, S. (1985). Issues in the study and application of social support. In Cohen, S. & Syme, S. (Eds). *Social Support and health.* Orlando: Academic Press.

Elal, G. & Krespi, M. (1999). Life events, social support and depression in hemodialysis patients. *Journal of Community and Applied Psychology, 9 (1),* 23-33.

Ellsion, C. E. & Taylor, R. J. (1996). Turning to prayer: Social and situational antecedents of religious coping among African-Americans. *Review of Religious Research, 38 (2),* 111-131.

Ferrans, C. & Powers, M. (1993). Quality of life of hemodialysis patients. *American Nephrology Nurses Association Journal, 20 (5),* 575-581.

Furr, L. A. (1998). Psycho-social aspects of serious renal disease and dialysis: A review of the literature. *Social Work in Health Care, 27* (3), 97-118.

Germain, C. & Bloom, M. (1999). *Human behavior and the social environment: An ecological view. Second edition.*

Harper, B. C. (1990). Blacks and the health care delivery system: Challenges and prospects. In Logan, S., Freeman, E. & Mcroy, R. (Eds). *Social work with Black families: A culturally specific perspective.* White Plains, NY: Longman.

Hill, R. (1972). *Strengths of Black families.* New York: National Urban League.

Hill, R. (1993). *Research on the African-American family: A holistic perspective.* Westport, CT: Auburn House.

Holder, B. (1997). Family support and survival among end-stage renal disease patients. *Advances in Renal Replacement Therapy, 4,* 13-21.

Kirst-Ashman, K. K. & Hull, G. H. (1999). *Understanding generalist practice: Second edition.* Chicago: Nelson-Hall.

Kutner, N. & Devins, G. (1998). A comparison of the quality of life reported by whites and elderly Blacks on dialysis. *Geriatric Nephrology and Urology, 8,* 77-83.

Leggat, J., Swartz, R. & Port, F. (1997). Withdrawl from dialysis: A review with an emphasis on the Black experience. *Advances in Renal Replacement Therapy, 4 (1),* 22-29.

Levin, J. S. (1996). How religion influences morbidity and health: Reflections on natural history, salutogenesis and host resistance. *Social Science and Medicine, 43 (5),* 849-864.

Levin, J. & Schiller, P. (1987). Is there a religious factor in health? *Journal of Religion and Health, 26,* 9-36.

Lewis, M. A., Rook, K. S. & Schwarzer, R. (1994). Social support, social control and health among the elderly. In Penhny, G. N., Bennett, P. & Herbert, M. (Eds). *Health psychology: A lifespan perspective.* Chur, Switzerland: Harwood Academic.

Littlejohn-Blake, S. & Darling, C. (1993). Understanding the strengths of African-American families. *Journal of Black Studies, 23 (4)*, 460-471.

Manns, W. (1997). Supportive roles of significant others in Black families. In Mcadoo, H. (Ed.). *Black families: Third edition.* Thousand Oaks: Sage Publications.

Mathews, D. (1998). Religion and spirituality in the care of patients with chronic renal failure. *Dialysis and Transplantation, 27 (3)*, 136-140.

McGee, H. & Bradley, C. (1994). Quality of life following renal failure: An introduction to the issues and challenges. In McGee, H. & Bradley, C. (Eds). *Quality of life following renal failure: Psychological challenges accompanying high technology medicine.* Switzerland: Harwood Academic.

Miller, S. D. (1993). Increasing the adjustment success of the disabled African-American. *Journal of Health & Social Policy, 5 (2)*, 87-104.

Neighbors, H. & Jackson, J. (1984). The use of informal and formal help: Patterns of illness behavior in the Black community. *American Journal of Community Psychology, 12 (6)*, 629-644.

Neighbors, H. & Jackson, J. (1996). Racism and the mental health of African-Americans: The role of self and system blame. *Ethnicity and Disease, 6 (1-2)*, 167-175.

Patterson, L. (1998). The philosophy and physics of holistic health care: Spiritual healing as a workable interpretation. *Journal of Advanced Nursing, 27*, 287-293.

Price, D. & Owen, W. (1997). African-Americans on maintenance dialysis: A review of racial differences in incidence, treatment and survival. *Advances in Renal Replacement Therapy, 4*, 3-12.

Raeburn, J. & Rootman, I. (1996). Quality of life and health promotion. In Renwick, R., Brown, I. & Nagler, M. (Eds.). *Quality of life in health promotion and rehabilitation: Conceptual approaches, issues and applications.* Thousand Oaks, CA: Sage Publications.

Reich, J., Erdal, K. & Zautra, A. (1997). Beliefs about control and health behaviors. In Gochman, D. (Ed). *Handbook of health behavior research I: Personal and social determinants.* New York: Plenum Press.

Saleeby, D. (1996). The strengths perspective in social work practice: Extensions and cautions. *Social Work, 41 (3)*, 296-305.

Skidmore, A., Thackery, M. & Farley, W. (1997). *Introduction to social work.* Boston: Allyn & Bacon.

Skinner, E. A. (1995). *Perceived control, motivation and coping.* Thousand Oaks, CA: Sage Publications.

Stack, C. (1974). *All our kin: Strategies for survival in a Black community.* New York: Harper & Row.

Taylor, R. & Chatters, L. (1991). Religious life. In Jackson, J. (Ed) *Family life in Black America* (pp. 105-123). Newbury Park: Sage Publications.

Taylor, R., Hardison, C. & Chatters, L. (1996). Kin and nonkin sources of informal assistance. In Neighbors, H. & Jackson, J. (Eds.). *Mental health in Black America.* Thousand Oaks, CA: Sage Publications.

Taylor, R., Jackson, J. & Chatters, L. (1997). *Family life in Black America.* Thousand Oaks, CA: Sage Publications.

Tell, G., Shumaker, S., Mittlemark, M., Russell, G., Hylander, B. & Burkhart, J. (1995). Social support and health-related quality of life in Black and white dialysis patients. *American Nephrology Nurses Association Journal, 22 (3)*, 301-308.

Tessaro, I., Eng, E. & Smith, J. (1994). Breast cancer screening in older African-American women: Qualitative research findings. *American Journal of Health Promotion, 8 (4),* 286-293.

Wallston, B., Wallston, K., Kaplan, G. & Maides, S. (1976). Development and validation of the health locus of control scales. *Journal of Consulting and Clinical Psychology, 44 (4), 580-585.*

Washington, A. W. (1999, June). *Cross cultural issues and adherence.* Paper presented at the meeting of the National Kidney Foundation-Clinical Nephrology Section. Washington, DC.

Motivated but Fearful:
Welfare Reform, Disability, and Race

Sandra Edmonds Crewe, PhD

SUMMARY. The Personal Responsibility and Work Opportunity Reconciliation Act (1996) instituted reforms in welfare that focused on mandatory work requirements. It imposes strict requirements and lifetime limits that force non-exempt individuals to work or risk sanctions. The law particularly impacts persons with disabilities because of the substantial numbers who believe they are unable to work. This article uses findings from a research study to discuss barriers faced by individuals with physical disabilities who are forced to find work under welfare reform. It highlights the experiences of African Americans who have the added burden of health disparities because of discriminatory and differential practices in diagnoses, treatment, access, and utilization. It also presents practice implications. *[Article copies available for a fee from The Haworth Document Delivery Service: 1-800-HAWORTH. E-mail address: <docdelivery@haworthpress. com> Website: <http:// www.HaworthPress.com> © 2002 by The Haworth Press, Inc. All rights reserved.]*

KEYWORDS. Welfare reform, disabilities, African Americans, health disparities

Sandra Edmonds Crewe is Assistant Professor, Howard University School of Social Work.

[Haworth co-indexing entry note]: "Motivated but Fearful: Welfare Reform, Disability, and Race." Crewe, Sandra Edmonds. Co-published simultaneously in *Journal of Health & Social Policy* (The Haworth Press, Inc.) Vol. 16, No. 1/2, 2002, pp. 55-68; and: *Disability and the Black Community* (ed: Sheila D. Miller) The Haworth Press, Inc., 2002, pp. 55-68. Single or multiple copies of this article are available for a fee from The Haworth Document Delivery Service [1-800-HAWORTH, 9:00 a.m. - 5:00 p.m. (EST). E-mail address: docdelivery@haworthpress.com].

10.1300/J045v16n01_06

INTRODUCTION

Individuals with disabilities represent one of the nation's most vulnerable populations. It is estimated that between 20% and 50% of welfare recipients have disabilities (Schroeder, 1999; Sweeney, 2000) and may risk benefit termination because of noncompliance or 60-month lifetime limits. Being aware of this possibility, critics of the 1996 Personal Responsibility and Work Opportunity Reconciliation Act (PRWORA) voiced strong concerns about the potential disparate effects of its mandatory work and time limits on vulnerable individuals including those with disabilities. Similarly, welfare reform critics raised concerns about the Temporary Assistance to Needy Families (TANF) program's potential predatory and disparate impact on African Americans who have higher rates of participation and disability caused by persistent racial discrimination that contributes to health disparities in the diagnoses, treatment, access, and utilization of services.

The National Association of Social Workers (NASW) states that the Americans with Disabilities Act (ADA) offers new civil rights yet provides little protection for the safety of the pensions and public welfare rights of persons with disabilities (2000). This harsh reality is evident under welfare reform in that many adults and children with disabilities are subject to benefit denial and termination. Thus, a major challenge for social workers is to merge the goals of self-sufficiency and civil rights for persons with disabilities. This is a daunting task, given the documented lack of cohesion between the two goals (O'Day, 1999; DeJong & Batavia, 1990).

Advocacy from the social work and allied professionals is needed to ensure that provisions are changed that place individuals with disabilities at risk of losing benefits and becoming further impoverished, stigmatized and disadvantaged. Limited attention, however, has been given to the multiple challenges of race and disability within the context of welfare reform. Using empirical research, this article examines welfare reform from the perspectives of physical disability and race. This dialogue is particularly relevant as we enter the post-authorization implementation of welfare reform. It offers empirical evidence that can assist local welfare offices in thier implementation of the 20% hardship exemption.

PRWORA AND PERSONS WITH DISABILITIES

The Personal Responsibility and Work Opportunity Reconciliation Act of 1996 (PL 104-103), known as the welfare reform law, is grounded in the conservative argument that the welfare system had created a culture of dependency and should be replaced with deterrent policies aimed at self-sufficiency (Jansson, 1997). A hallmark of this law was the repeal of the Aid to Families with Dependent Children (AFDC) entitlement program and the creation of the block granted Temporary Assistance to Needy Families (TANF) program (Office of Civil Rights, 2001; Zastrow, 2000; Personal Responsibility, 1996). Simply stated, welfare reform fostered local programs defined by "work first" and "lifetime limits."

Welfare roll declines also raise important questions about the well-being outcomes of persons once they leave. Nationwide "leaver" studies provide some added insight. According to the Urban Institute's (1999) national study, *Work Activity and Obstacles to Work Among TANF Recipients,* 25% of current recipients reported poor general health as a key reason for not working (Zedlewski, 1999). Numerous state studies also confirm that substantial numbers of parents who claim disabilities are being terminated from TANF (Sweeney, 2000). Four years after the implementation of PRWORA, U.S. Representative Stephen Horn stated that almost 75% of working age adults with disabilities are not working or underemployed (Horn, 2000). He noted that persons with disabilities needed extra attention in the nation's welfare to work effort. The U.S. Department of Health and Human Services Office of Civil Rights (OCR) also recognized the need for guidance to TANF agencies and issued policy guidance to avoid "over sanction" of individuals where sanctions are inappropriate (Office of Civil Rights, 2001). The guidance clarified the obligation of Title II of the ADA and Section 504 regarding the implementation of welfare reform. It emphasized the needs of a cohort of families with multiple barriers who "due to known or unrecognized disabilities, need additional training, accommodations, and support services to prepare for or succeed at work" (p. 4).

The Center on Budget and Policy Priorities' (Sweeney, 2000) study on welfare recipients with disabilities documents that "a significant portion of parents who receive TANF or who have left TANF have disabilities or health conditions that may affect their ability to succeed in the workplace without appropriate supports and services to help them address barriers" (p. 2). The study reports that between one-fifth and one-half of non-working TANF recipients have health problems that they believe keep them from working. At the end of fiscal year 1999, only 14% of work exemptions were granted for persons with disabilities. Yet, among former non-working TANF recipients, one-fifth to two-fifths claim an inability to work due to disability, health condition, or illness (Sweeney, 2000). These data further underscore the importance of examining the policy implications of welfare reform for persons with disabilities.

The U.S. Department of Health and Human Services, Administration for Children and Families (ACF) indicate African American families represent the largest segment (38.6%) of families receiving TANF (ACF, 2000). This places them at greater risk of lifetime sanctions. In fact, data from the U.S. Department of Health and Human Services indicate that three out of five TANF adult recipients are members of minority or ethnic groups (ACF, 2000). The picture is even more revealing when the evaluation compares the experiences of urban agencies with large concentrations of African Americans to their contiguous suburban agencies (Meyers, 2001).

CONCEPTUAL FRAMEWORK

The bodies of literature on welfare reform and persons with disabilities reflect the paramount importance of a conceptual framework that can explain human behavior in the context of the environment. Success in moving from welfare to work is inextricably related to how well individuals access systems and how well systems respond to individual needs. Studies have demonstrated that persons with disabilities have experienced more difficulties in participating in required work activities because of a health or emotional problem (Stapleton et al., 1995). Furthermore, Stapleton et al. (1995) report that distinguishing features of successful programs include a comprehensive range of services that are individually tailored to meet each client's specific needs and goals. Understanding the path to self-sufficiency or work requires an understanding of the individual's abilities and barriers related to maximizing their abilities. The interaction of person in environment is particularly important in studying this group because the environment often determines whether individuals are able to overcome the emotional and physical challenges posed by their disability. The ecosystem perspective is especially valuable in examining the welfare reform experience of persons with disabilities because it can help social workers arrange, integrate, and systematize knowledge about how people interrelate with each other and with their environments (Pillari & Newsome, 1998). It is a conceptual framework that considers the layers of interactions in explaining human behavior and avoids the devaluing of the individual by equating her with her disability (Michilin & Juarez-Marazzo, 2001). The ecosystems perspective integrates the ecology and general systems theory and posits, "seeing people in their ecological milieu and in their transactions lets us assess their strengths and weaknesses in their own physical, psychological, and social environments" (Pillari & Newsome, p. 19). Additionally, the ecological perspective addresses adaptive functioning capacities and stress reactions and acknowledges the unequal power arrangements and internalized oppression (Worden, 2001).

Cultural-duality theory also helps to order the knowledge related to the influence of race on persons with disabilities. The ramifications of physical disabilities on individuals and their transactions are expansive, convoluted, and confounded by being a member of an oppressed or minority group (Michilin & Juarez-Marazzo, 2001). According to Chestang, the socio-environmental conditions of social injustice, social inconsistency, and personal impotence influence social functioning of African Americans and other minority groups (Lum, 2000). The cultural-duality theory holds that the historical disparate treatment of African Americans results in them using the dominant culture to gain access to material goods/programs and their nurturing community to fulfill needs of psychological, emotional, and social support (Chestang, 1976).

RESEARCH STUDY

This research sought to identify characteristics of a sample of 268 households in an urban county remaining on the TANF rolls two years after the implementation of the Personal Responsibility and Work Opportunity Reconciliation Act. Additionally, it investigated the personal and systemic barriers that they were experiencing in moving from welfare to work. The clients were classified, using hierarchal cluster analysis, into seven clusters of risks based upon selected factors. The seven clusters are based upon their dominant characteristics listed in Table 1. This article examines more closely health and disability findings through analysis of characteristics of 28 respondents to the 200 mailed surveys who identified physical disability as an important reason for not working full time. Table 1 includes the dominant characteristics of the seven clusters including the health and disability cluster (Crewe, Schervish & Gourdine, 2000). Sixty-five percent of clients who fall into the health and disability risk cluster report health problems and almost 61% have physical disabilities. The article also focuses on the differences imposed by the cumulative disadvantage of race and disability.

RESEARCH RESULTS

" *[My] legs and lower back give out, diabetes is out of control, [I have] infections every other month.*" Like this TANF recipient, 14% (n = 28) of the sample reported a physical disability as their reason for not working. Additionally 20% (n = 40) reported not working because of health problems. Although there is a significant relationship using chi square (p = .00) between not working due to physical disability and not working because of health problems, the analyses

TABLE 1. Risk Clusters

	Cluster*						
	1	2	3	4	5	6	7
	High Risk	Education & Training	Health & Mental Health	Violence, Victimization & Education	Housing	Health & Disability	Child Care, Transportation & Other
% in each cluster	33.7	14.6	10.1	9.5	7.5	13.6	11.1
Clustering Factor							
Violence in the home	35			30		0	
Homeless in past year	50	0	0	0	50	0	0
Depression	29.5		23.1				
Not enough food		28.1			26.3		
Lack of permanent housing	50				19.2		
No child care	24						32
No transportation	14.5			21			17.7
Physical disability	25	0				60.7	0
Lack of skills	26.7	26.7		18.3			
Lack of education	22.7	31.8		18.2			
Can't get hired	21.1	60.5	0		0		
Health problems	27.5			0	0	65	0
Need license or certificate	31.8	22.7		27.3			
Lack of experience	21	35.5		24.2			
Don't understand rules	0	0	0	0	0	100	0
No one is helping	33.3	47.6					0
Pay is too low	28.6			36.7			0
Other reasons	37						44.4

*Percent of those indicating having the problem, distributed across clusters.

are restricted to the clients who specifically stated a physical disability as a barrier to their working (see Table 2).

The sample is 96% female and 81% African American. The mean age is 36.4 years (median 38 years) of age as compared with a mean age of 32.3 years (median 31 years) for individuals in the sample not identifying a disability. Almost 58% are single and 38.4% are divorced or separated. This compares with 86.5% and 9.8%, respectively, among the non-disabled respondents. Just over 53% have a high school diploma and almost 11% report some college. This re-

TABLE 2. Selected Comparisons of TANF Clients Based on Disability Status

SELECTED VARIABLES	PHYSICAL DISABILITIES n = 28	WITHOUT PHYSICAL DISABILITIES n = 171
	Percentage	Percentage
Age (mean years)	36.4	32.3
Race		
African American	80.8	95.5
White	19.0	4.5
Education		
High School Diploma	53.6	39.3
Some College	11.0	16.7
Welfare Dependency Spells		
Five or more years	50.0	41.6
Understand Changes	29.6	41.4
Thinks she can do what is asked*	56.0	80.2
Not Employed	86.0	59.0
Experienced depression past year	32.1	40.4
Worship Attendance (weekly)	39.3	28.5
Reasons Not Working		
Not Motivated	3.6	.6
Discrimination	7.1	2.9
No Child Care	17.9	26.3
No Transportation	32.1	31.0
Mental Disability	10.7	2.3
Not Enough Education	7.1	24.6
Not Enough Skills	28.6	30.4
Health Problems*	64.3	12.9
Feelings About Finding Work		
Will find in next six months*	7.1	20.5
Discouraged	21.4	9.4
Afraid/Frightened *	28.6	9.9
Angry/resentful	10.7	7.6

* $p = < .05$

flects a higher educational level than the non-disabled respondents, 39% of whom have high school diplomas and 16.7% some college. Consistently, the data show that 7.1% of persons with disabilities as compared to 24.6% of others indicate insufficient education as a contributing factor to their not working. The persons with disabilities report higher weekly church attendance (39%) than do individuals not reporting a physical disability (28.5%).

The cohort reporting physical disabilities also has been on welfare longer than their counterparts. Fifty percent have received assistance for five or more years as compared to 41.6% of the non-disabled group. Fewer individuals (29.6%) with physical disabilities report that they understand the welfare changes than do individuals who did not report a disability (41.4%). Consistent with the literature, almost 86% of persons with physical disabilities as compared with 59% of non-disabled persons had not found employment since the implementation of welfare reform. However, only 3.6% of persons with disabilities state that they were not motivated to find work. The data show that 7% of persons with disabilities as compared to just over 1% of the non-disabled group state that they don't understand the rules. Within this cluster, 100% do not understand the rules. This confirms the earlier finding regarding their difficulty in understanding and carrying out what is expected of them.

Thinking about the next six months, almost 93% of persons with physical disabilities as compared with 80% of non-disabled clients did *not* feel optimistic about finding work (p = .03). Although not optimistic, most (over 80%) are *not* discouraged, angry or resentful about having to find work. However, individuals with physical disabilities are more likely than non-disabled respondents to be fearful and afraid of not finding work (p = .01). They also exhibit low self-efficacy. When compared to non-disabled clients, they do not feel that they can do what is expected of them (p = .01). In their own words TANF clients speak of their disabilities.

- *July 23, 1999, I had lung surgery, [I] can't breathe too good . . . I am on oxygen and take three different inhalers every three hours.*
- *[I have] a medical problem with my feet that causes me to not be able to do no type of weight bearing on any job for no long period of time.*
- *I have diabetes which keep me sometime not feeling well.*

Their words add depth by speaking to their lived-experiences and offer explanation for their low self-efficacy. Their self-identified medical conditions document barriers to obtaining many of the traditional entry level (minimum wage) positions that are available to individuals moving from welfare to work. Despite their problems, they remain relatively optimistic and report lower levels of depression than individuals who did not report a physical disability.

DISCUSSION

Prior to the 1996 PRWORA, it was known that substantial numbers of welfare recipients, approximately 20%, were disabled (Adler, 1993). Perhaps this estimate was used to determine the 20% hardship exemption and provide the "safety net" to protect those who were unable to work. It appears, however, that the safety net is not effective for all who require special assistance. With the tremendous pressure to move families off welfare, it is possible that the needs of individuals with disabilities are sometimes overlooked, ignored, or simply not understood. It is all too possible that some persons with disabilities were included in a group assumed to be seeking "asylum" from work because of a basic lack of motivation to work. On the other hand, it is highly possible that persons who claimed disabilities were assumed to be individuals who could not work rather than individuals requiring strategic supports to enable them to work successfully.

The research is particularly valuable in pointing out the cohort of clients who consider themselves physically unable to work but are required to under TANF rules. According to the data, 85% have applied for other financial benefits including 32% who have applied for disability under Social Security or SSI. This compares to just over 5% of the non-disabled group. Equally important is that although they report that their physical disability is a primary cause for them not working, 18% have been denied coverage and 58% are waiting for a decision. Those who have been denied disability coverage are indeed at high risk of losing benefits unless safeguards are put in place to assist them in locating employment that is respectful of their physical needs or they receive assistance in validating their physical impairment. Whether this happens is largely dependent upon the attitude and preparation of front line workers to address the needs of persons with disabilities.

The data on the number of sanctioned TANF families who claim disabilities presents documentation that persons reporting health problems are more likely to be sanctioned. Why? This is a compelling question that demands an examination of policies regarding sanctioning persons who feel that they are unable to work due to physical limitations. Another red herring identified by this study is that individuals with disabilities report lesser understanding of the welfare changes than do others. Previous research has linked low self-esteem and self-efficacy with expected difficulty in complying with expanded and stricter work requirements (Kunz & Kalil, 1999). The research on sanctions also confirms that lack of understanding of program requirements is another factor associated with higher levels of sanctioning. For example, Sweeney (2000) reports that in Delaware sanctioned families with health problems were more likely to experience difficulty in understanding TANF rules. Similarly, 28% of sanctioned Iowa's participants with health problems reported a lack of understanding of the program requirements (Sweeney, 2000). This study confirmed these findings in that only 30% of the respondents indicated that they understood the welfare rules "very well."

While race is important, the study shows that persons with disabilities are more alike than different. However, race does matter. The study uncovers some differences that suggest that the cumulative disadvantage of discriminatory practices as well as their access to resources influence the outcomes of African American persons with disabilities. The omens of premature or unfair benefit termination are even more pronounced for African Americans who are often disadvantaged by discrimination in the job market. In her book, *"No Shame in My Game: The Working Poor in the Inner City,"* Katherine Newman (1999, p. 223) states that "race heightens the stresses of poverty, especially when a tightening job market forces minorities of all colors into a scramble for the share of the shrinking pie." Considering that the research has documented that understanding the rules, mental health, longevity on welfare, and mental health are indicators of high risk for termination (Sweeney, 2000), African Americans with disabilities are at higher risk than their White counterparts.

The study documents that African Americans report lower levels of understanding of the rules, longer spells on welfare, and higher rates of depression. Additionally, they report less support from the local welfare office and more help from families and outside sources (Crewe, 1997; Gooden, 1998, 1999, 2000). This is consistent with Chestang's cultural duality theory (Chestang, 1976; Lum, 2000). Initial criticism of welfare reform by African Americans was in part based upon the concern of disparate treatment and the legacy of broken promises and history replete with well-intended failed social experiments (Jeff, 1997; Million Family March, 2000). This criticism was grounded in the belief that federal policy discussions about welfare reform deliberately shifted the focus from the structural constraints to one that unfairly targeted recipient behavior change (Staples, 1997; Yoo, 1999). Findings from this study invite further examination of disparities in policy implementation attributed to race and disability.

CONCLUSIONS AND IMPLICATIONS
FOR POLICY AND PRACTICE

The *NASW Policy Statement on TANF: Welfare Reform*, states that the social work profession has the responsibility to "identify propaganda and misinformation from all quarters and to provide accurate and relevant information about the reality of poverty, the history of social policy on poverty and impact of these policies on vulnerable groups" (NASW, 2000, p. 297). This research and a review of the literature document that persons with health disabilities are vulnerable to termination of benefits because of sanctions, inability to complete work activities, and lifetime limits. In order to survive welfare reform they need assistance in understanding the rules, their rights, the opportunities, and the support systems. Ironically, frontline workers are also victimized by welfare reform. They are asked to make tough calls and issue sanctions in situations that they have neither the appropriate time nor training to complete professional assessments. A social work client advocate observed that sometimes workers follow the rules and end up "dis-enabling" rather than enabling the person.

The current delivery system must use the evidence that shows disparate treatment on the basis of race and disability and craft "real" safety nets and install checkpoints to ensure that individuals who exit the system get what they need to survive and thrive. Most importantly, there must be a conscientious effort to root out the notion that many persons who claim physical disabilities are motivated by a desire to manipulate the system and avoid work. The evidence does not support a desire to abuse the system; therefore, we must use the evidence to address this misconception. Similarly, the evidence suggests that effective practice with African Americans requires an awareness of the cumulative effects of racism and denied or deferred opportunities and rights.

As we enter the post-reauthorization cycle of PRWORA, empirical evidence that adds to our understanding of the cumulative effect of health disparities of African Americans and other minority TANF recipients must become a higher priority. If we are to allay their fears, more research is critically needed that gives a voice to those who are disempowered and made vulnerable by the multiple risks imposed by poverty, race, and gender. The evidence is that persons with disabilities are disproportionally leaving the rolls and not working. There is disparity in perceived access to supports based upon race. The 20% hardship exemption is inadequate for some jurisdictions. Worker discretion creates disparity based upon race. People are afraid because they don't believe they can do what is expected. Most want to work. They have strengths. They need help and understanding. They need us to listen. In closing, the words from a TANF client poignantly address the need for understanding, compassion, and support in the implementation of welfare reform for persons with disabilities. *"I think it's good that you help people like myself find a good job, but in my case, my health won't allow me to do nothing. I'm deeply sorry, but I can't help it. Please understand."*

REAUTHORIZATION REFERENCES

Greenberg, M. (2002). Bush's blunder. *The American Prospect*, 13 (13). Available online <*http://www.clasp.org/DMS/Documents/10224427766.57/greenberg-m.html*>.
Whitehouse (2002, February 26). President announces welfare reform agenda. Retrieved March 02, 2002 from <*http://www.whitehouse.gov/news/releases/ 2002/02/ print/20020226-11.html*>.
Whitehouse (2002). Working Toward Independence. Retrieved March 02, 2002 from <*http://www.whitehouse.gov/news/releases/2002/02/welfarereform-announcement-book.pdf*>.

REFERENCES

Adler, M. (1993). Disability among women on AFDC: An issue revisited. Office of the Assistant Secretary for Planning and Evaluation, U.S. Department of Health and Human Services. Available online at *<http://www.aspe.hhs.gov/daltcp/reports/afdcwomn.htm>*.

Administration for Children and Families (ACF) (2000). *Characteristics and financial circumstances of TANF recipients–Fiscal year 1999*. (U.S. Department of Health and Human Services, Act, Office of Planning Research and Evaluation). Available online at *<http://www.acf.dhhs.gov/programs/opre/characteristics/fy99/analysis.htm>*.

American with Disabilities Act of 1990, P.L. 101-336, 104 Stat. 327.

Ayres-Williams, R. & Graves, N. (1998). Challenged but not disabled. *Black Enterprise, 28*(7) Available online EBSCO Host.

Chestang, L. (1976). Environmental influences on social functioning: The black experience. In P. San Juan Cafferty & L. Chestang (Eds.), *The diverse society: Implications for social policy* (pp. 59-74). Washington, DC: National Association of Social Workers.

Clinton, W. (1996). Statement on welfare reform. Weekly Compilation of Presidential Documents, 8/5/96, vol. 32, issue 31, pp. 1353.

Crewe, S.E. (1997). *Unmotivated or unchallenged: An ethnographic study of sanctioned welfare recipients residing in federally assisted housing.* Unpublished doctoral dissertation, Howard University, Washington, DC.

Crewe, S.E., Schervish, P., & Gourdine, R.M. (2000). *Welfare reform: Risk and resilience indicators of TCA customers in Prince George's County, Maryland.* Howard University E. Franklin Frazier Research Center, Washington, DC.

DeJong, G. & Batavia, A. (1999). The Americans with Disabilities Act and the current state of U.S. disability policy. *Journal of Disability Policy Studies 1*(3), 65-74.

Gooden, S.T. (1998). All things not being equal: Differences in caseworker support toward Black and White welfare clients. *Harvard Journal of African Americans Public Policy*, vol. 4.

Gooden, S.T. (1999). Welfare recipients' experiences with employers. *Journal of Public Management and Social Policy, 5*(1).

Gooden, S.T. (2000). Examining employment outcomes of White and Black welfare recipients. *Journal of Poverty*, 4 (3), pp. 21-41.

Horn, S. (2000). The Pride of self-sufficiency. *Press Release,* August 30, 2000. FDCH Press Releases eMediaMillWorks, Inc., Washington, DC.

Jansson, B.S. (1997). The reluctant welfare state. Pacific Cole, CA.: Brooks-Cole Publishing Company.

Jeff, M.X. (1997). The National Association of Black Social Workers' reflection on the new welfare reform law. *Harvard Journal of African American Public Policy*, pp. 49-58.

Kunz, J. & Kalil, A. (1999). Self esteem, self-efficacy, and welfare use. *Social Work Research, 23*(2), pp. 119-126.

Lum, D. (2000). *Social work practice and people of color.* Belmont, CA: Brooks Cole Publishing.

Meadows, M. (1999). Improving the quality of life for minorities with disabilities. *Closing the Gap*. Newsletter. Office of Minority Health, Office of Public Health and Science, U.S. Department of Health and Human Services, October/November 1999 (pp. 1-2).

Meyers, C.S. (2001). The District and Baltimore face double whammy in welfare reform: Greater challenges and less funding for needed services. Washington, DC: The Brookings Institution. Available online *<http://www.brook.edu/es/urban/gwrp/welfare _double_whammy_fullreport.htm>*.

Michilin, P. & Juarez-Marazzo, S. (2001). Ablelism: Social work practice with individuals with physical disabilities. In G.A. Appleby, E. Colon, & J. Hamilton (Eds.), *Diversity, oppression, and social functioning: Person-in-environment assessment an intervention* (pp. 179-194). Boston: Allyn & Bacon.

Million Family March (2000). *The National agenda: Public policy issues, analyses, and programmatic plan of action 2000-2008*. Washington, DC: Author.

National Association of Social Workers (2000). Social work speaks: NASW policy statements 2000-2003. Washington, DC: Author.

Newman, K. (1999). *No shame in my game: The working poor in the inner city*. New York:Vintage Books.

O'Day, B. (1999). Policy barriers for people with disabilities who want to work. *American Rehabilitation*, vol. 25, 1, 8-16.

Office of Civil Rights (2001). Prohibition against discrimination on the basis of disability in the administration of TANF. Available on line *<http://www.hhs.gov/ocr/prohibition.html>*.

Personal Responsibility and Work Opportunity Reconciliation Act of 1996, P.L. 104-193, 110 Stat. 2105.

Pillari, V. & Newsome, M. (1998). *Human behavior in the social environment: Families, groups, organizations and communities*. Pacific Grove, CA: Brooks/Cole Publishing.

Ross, H. (1999). President's Committee addresses unemployment. *Closing the Gap*. Newsletter. Office of Minority Health, Office of Public Health and Science, U.S. Department of Health and Human Services, October/November 1999 (p. 11).

Schroeder, F. (1999). Welfare reform: Linking TANF and VR. American Rehabilitation, vol. 25, 1.

Staples, R. (1999). *The Black family: Essays and studies* (6th ed.). Belmont, CA: Wadsworth Publishing Company.

Stapleton, D, Alecxih, L., Barnow, B., Coleman, K., Livermore, G., Lo, G., Lutsky, S, & Zeuschner, A. (1995). An exploratory study of barriers and incentives to improving labor participation among persons with significant disabilities. Available online *<http://www.aspe.hhs.gov/daqltcp/reports/explores.htm>*.

Sweeney, E.P. (2000). Recent studies indicate that many parents who are current or former welfare recipients have disabilities or other medial conditions. Available online *<http://www.cbpp.org/2-29-00wel.htm>*.

U.S. Department of Commerce, Bureau of the Census (1999). Labor force status and other characteristics of persons with a work disability. Washington, DC: US Government Printing Office.

U.S. Department of Health and Human Services (2000). HHS Fact Sheet: HHS Strategies for improving minority health. Washington: DC. Author available on line *<http://waisgate.hhs.gov/cgi-bin/>*.

Worden, B. (2001). Women and sexist oppression. In G.A. Appleby, E. Colon, and J. Hamilton (Eds.), *Diversity, oppression, and social functioning: Person-in-environment assessment and intervention* (pp. 70-91). Boston: Allyn & Bacon.

Yoo, G.J. (1999). Racial inequality. Welfare reform and Black families: The 1996 Personal Responsibility and Work Opportunity Reconciliation Act. In R. Staples (Ed.), *The Black family* (pp. 357-366). Belmont, CA: Wadsworth Publishing Company.

Zastrow, C. (2000). *Introduction to social work and social welfare.* Belmont, CA: Wadsworth Publishing Company.

Zedlewski, S. (1999). Work activity and obstacles to work among TANF recipients, Urban Institute, Series B., No. B-2, September 1999. Available online <*http://www.newfederalism. urban.org/html/series_b/b2/anf_b2.html*>.

Predicting Weekly Earning
for Consumers with Severe Disabilities:
Implications for Welfare Reform
and Vocational Rehabilitation

Ted M. Daniels, MBA, MA
Elijah Mickel, DSW, CRT, LICSW

SUMMARY. This 1999 research analyzed selected descriptive variables for consumers with significant disabilities, who were successfully employed. The goal was to investigate employment outcomes for consumers whose cases were closed as successfully employed. Human capital theory provided the theoretical underpinnings for evaluating the findings. This study empirically assessed factors which contributed to increased weekly earnings for consumers of state vocational rehabilitation services with severe disabilities. The variables included in this study were weekly earnings at closure, correlated with year last employed, highest grade completed, and birth year. The study found that 17.2% of variability in weekly earnings of the significantly disabled consumers can be predicted by these variables. Education, age, and work experience were found to be predictors of potential earning power. These findings can be used to provide the foundation for the development of reliable

---

Ted M. Daniels is Deputy Administrator, D. C. Department of Vocational Rehabilitation. Elijah Mickel is Professor, Delaware State University.

[Haworth co-indexing entry note]: "Predicting Weekly Earning for Consumers with Severe Disabilities: Implications for Welfare Reform and Vocational Rehabilitation." Daniels, Ted, M., and Elijah Mickel. Co-published simultaneously in *Journal of Health & Social Policy* (The Haworth Press, Inc.) Vol. 16, No. 1/2, 2002, pp. 69-79; and: *Disability and the Black Community* (ed: Sheila D. Miller) The Haworth Press, Inc., 2002, pp. 69-79. Single or multiple copies of this article are available for a fee from The Haworth Document Delivery Service [1-800-HAWORTH, 9:00 a.m. - 5:00 p.m. (EST). E-mail address: docdelivery@haworthpress.com].

10.1300/J045v16n01_07

program evaluation as well as clinical interventions. This study links outcomes to the services provided. It further provides the data necessary to support policy development in the areas of rehabilitation and welfare reform. *[Article copies available for a fee from The Haworth Document Delivery Service: 1-800-HAWORTH. E-mail address: <docdelivery@haworthpress. com> Website: <http://www.HaworthPress.com> © 2002 by The Haworth Press, Inc. All rights reserved.]*

KEYWORDS. Age, African American, disabilities, education, employment, policy, TANF (Temporary Assistance for Needy Families), vocational rehabilitation, weekly earnings, welfare reform, work

INTRODUCTION

This article is based upon an empirical study of persons with severe disabilities. It evaluates the contributions of age, education and employment. It is through an understanding of the interplay of these and other variables that one can begin, based upon empirical data, to understand the possible outcome of the focus on employment in the welfare reform system. The outcome of this study can be a harbinger for understanding the possible long-term impact of welfare reform. The data contains relevant characteristics which can aid in futuristic speculation which is empirically grounded.

The Rehabilitation Services Administration (RSA) population is one that has been oppressed and discounted in a capitalistic society. Since the birth of this nation, persons with disabilities have been among the most disenfranchised segment of the population (Williamson, 1998; and Wright, 1960). Governmental statistics show that persons with significant disabilities are the least educated, the most likely to be unemployed and, as they get older, the least likely to obtain an occupation which pays a living wage (www.census.gov, 1995). African Americans have been even more discriminated against based upon both disability (Dunham, Holliday, Douget, Koller, Presberry, and Wooderson, 1998) and racial discrimination (Adams, 2001; Akabas and Gates, 1997; and Belgrave and Walker, 1991). A majority of the sample used in this study are African Americans. Correlating the Anderson Model (accessibility, availability, affordability, and acceptability) with the construct of racism can provide a set of interrelated propositions to explain these phenomena (Proctor and Stiffman, 1998). Many have been recipients of income maintenance and most have been thrust into the capitalist system at the pre-blue collar employment level. This data provides the possible future outcome for the nonsubsidized income maintenance recipient.

The stigma associated with receiving many forms of welfare is similar to that for people with disability. Employment rates for people with disabilities are lowest of many groups which makes their full participation in the society difficult. Therefore, the reentry process for the RSA population mirrors the process of reentry of welfare leavers into a working society. Work provides financial means for participation and accords status, and provides an environment where one can build friendships and community connections. It further undergirds the health and economy of the U.S.

An investigation of level of education and other predictors of weekly earnings was expected to add to the knowledge in the area of empirical research and provide some basis for social work and rehabilitation policy and practice reform. This research is necessary to improve outcomes of rehabilitation services administration. As we move into the 21st century accountability and performance measures are increasingly more commonplace. Administrative decisions are increasingly informed by data, and sophisticated program evaluation systems provide an empirical foundation. There is a dearth of empirical data in this area. According to GAO (1996, p. 22), "Most of the 26 employment focused programs we examined have not been formally evaluated. . . . For some of the programs that did collect outcome data, the information collected was not sufficient to adequately link outcomes to the services provided." Social systems are making rapid, yet informed adjustments while organizations develop the capacity to learn what works. Information systems provide feedback necessary to assess performance and learn from experiences. An examination of predictors of earnings for rehabilitation clients is postulated to provide insights for practitioners, administrators, policy makers, and consumers of services.

WELFARE REFORM

The framers of the Personal Responsibility and Work Opportunity Reconciliation Act of 1996 (PRWORA) made legislative changes based upon the value of work as the answer to economic exclusion. States were required to document work participation of increasing shares of its caseload. These changes were implemented under the provisions of Temporary Assistance for Needy Families (TANF). The most significant component of welfare reform was the requirement to work, as noted by Zedlewski, Holcomb and Duke (1998, p. 30). It is "States must include all families with adults in their work participation rates unless the family has a child under age one. All welfare recipients not exempt from work participation must be in a work activity by the end of two years to continue receiving assistance." Although work for some recipients of public assistance has not been ignored there has been a portion of the recipient population considered either difficult or unlikely to be placed in jobs. This population has been considered employment unable.

The service provider's role is one of facilitating reengagement in the capital-labor paradigm. Employment is the objective, although a livable wage may not be the outcome. According to Brauner and Loprest (1999, p. 6), "Wisconsin . . . calculated how actual earnings after leaving welfare compared with the poverty level, taking into account the number of children. The study found that for leavers who did not return to welfare, a little more than a third to about half of leavers' earnings were above the poverty level, depending on the number of children." By inference this data suggests that the majority of leavers are employed as unskilled labor.

The public welfare system under welfare reform has reengaged itself as a tool of capitalism to provide the basic labor component that is the pre-blue collar worker–unskilled and uneducated. The underemployed worker is the one who provides the fodder for the service industry. According to Brauner and Loprest (1999, p. 9), "Information on wages, earnings and type of job reveals that leavers usually have low-wage jobs, so their earnings remain low despite high employment rates and number of hours worked. The earnings information gathered from these studies shows that the average leaver's earnings are below the poverty level, and most leavers report having incomes that are lower than or similar to their combined earnings and benefits before exit."

The PRWORA of 1996 has been in effect long enough for a number of evaluations to be conducted(Green, Boots and Tumlin, 1999; Zedlewski, Holcomb and Duke, 1998). In addition, Brauner and Loprest (1999, p. 1) report "From March 1994 (the peak for welfare caseloads) to September 1998, the national case load of Aid to Families with Dependent Children (AFDC, now called Temporary Assistance for Needy Families–TANF) decreased by 43 percent. Many states' caseloads fell even more; for example, Wisconsin's caseload decreased by 87 percent, South Carolina's by 61 percent, and Texas's by 55 percent." This data provided a glimpse of what may potentially be the major short-term outcomes of this altered system. Long-term, without subsidized employment, outcomes are speculative at best (Lerman, Loprest and Ratcliffe, 1999).

The PRWORA of 1996 has altered the relationship between the consumer and the income maintenance system. It changed the income maintenance system from a system that provided direct sustenance, to alleviate a lack of resources, to one that focuses upon providing a gateway to employability (Coe, Acs, Lerman and Watson, 1998). It has also altered the role from consumer to one of potential human capital. The consumer is viewed as pre-capital-labor in a temporary state of nonengagement.

HUMAN CAPITAL THEORY

The theoretical framework for this research study is premised on the human capital theory. Essentially, vocational rehabilitation services involve a consumer who makes "informed choices" concerning investment(s) which build human capital. The mission of the public vocational rehabilitation program is to provide resources and identify opportunities, such as education, for eligible persons with disabilities to enter or reenter the work force. According to Brookins (1998, p. 1), "The term human capital" is a familiar one to economists. The concept emerged in the late 1950s at the University of Chicago as a set of labor economics theories that could explain and predict the relative productivity of individuals. In its most basic sense, human capital theory posits that individuals possess a stock of skills acquired through investments, such as in education and training. This stock is the sum of acquired skills (minus their depreciation depending on market demands, societal forces, and other factors) and is generally related to a person's earnings. The greater the human capital, theory suggests, the higher an individual's earnings.

Human capital theory could well be the foundation for welfare reform and the public vocational rehabilitation program. To the extent that decisions during stages of the life cycle (starting at adolescence) reduce the investment, they reduce human capital and future earnings (Parkman, 1992; and Becker, 1964). Generally, the vocational rehabilitation worker initiates acquisition of the consumers' choice(s) of products and services. To prepare for employment, the consumer may decide, as part of his/her employment plan, to seek vocational skills training, participate in on-the-job training, pursue an associates, a bachelors or graduate degree. If the consumer chooses neither and opts to forgo some form of education in favor of direct job placement, he/she loses the opportunity to make an investment towards accumulating human capital, which leads to higher earnings for persons participating in the work force.

The connections among length of time absent from the labor force or, in this case years since last employed, is another aspect of human capital theory. A number of theories have been put forth to describe the relationships among level of education and other characteristics with earnings (Gittleman, 1994). Human capital theory asserts that levels of experience are similar to levels of education, as a predictor variable for levels of earnings. Specifically, human capital theory asserts that with additional labor market experience, individuals will receive more on-the-job training, and the skills developed in this process will enable them to eventually receive higher earnings. As it relates to age, human capital theory asserts that older workers may not be much different from younger workers. Older workers have more opportunities to have higher earnings, all other variables held constant, for several reasons, including seniority provisions in occupations.

One's human capital is acquired and maintained through investment and is based on her/his potential earnings. Most persons with disabilities are among the least likely to be employed; the most likely to be recipients of public support; the most likely to be classified as poor. They are the most likely to require specialized services for job placement assistance; and for those who become employed, the most likely to be underemployed, the most likely to be working in a part-time job and the group with the lowest level of earnings (Gittleman, 1994). This profile is one that closely matches those who leave the welfare system through employment.

METHOD

The question this study posed to answer was whether a significant relationship existed between selected variables (age, education, and last year employed) and successful employment outcomes as measured by weekly earnings at case closure. This research study was designed to evaluate if selected variables could predict weekly earnings as an employment outcome for consumers whose cases were closed as successfully employed. Increased attention to the earnings of consumers closed in status 26 (rehabilitated) is precipitated by the increasing awareness that though placed in employment as successfully rehabilitated, consumers may not be earning sufficient income to sustain themselves above the poverty level. The objective of this study was to find the predictors of successful employment outcomes for the population identified as significantly disabled by a vocational rehabilitation program.

This research study evaluated level of education, time since last employed, and age as predictors of "level of earnings" of persons with significant disabilities. Significantly disabled clients are those with a significant physical or mental disability whose case has been coded in all of the "Significantly Disabled Coding Series" (e.g.,100, 200, 300, 400, 500, 600, and 700) in the RSA disability coding system. The successfully closed cases of three hundred and seventy-four clients (N = 374) of a major northeastern city's vocational rehabilitation agency were used in the study. The Rehabilitation Services Administration (RSA), were one of 82 State-Federal Vocational Rehabilitation Programs in the United States.

The population for this study comprised all status 26 consumers placed in competitive employment by a state-federal vocational rehabilitation (VR) program. A status 26 is the closure of a consumer's case after placement in competitive employment and maintaining the job for a minimum of 60 days following the date entering the job. A purposive sample of data for this population were taken from the cumulative caseload report for fiscal year 1998.

The present study used the most recent year for which data was available–the fiscal year 1998, which included data for 1435 closed cases. After case selecting the participants, 665 status 26 "rehabilitated," closed cases were identified. From this number (n = 665), further re-coding was done to only include consumers who were identified as Significantly Disabled (SD) and placed in competitive employment. This selection resulted in 443 cases. Of the 443 cases 236 were male and 207 were female. Thirty-two respondents were of Hispanic origin, 59 were white, eight were Asian or Pacific Islander and 376 were Black. The final number of cases usable for the present study was 374. The design of this study is an ex post facto with exploratory objectives. Analysis of variable began with descriptive statistics to determine if a relationship existed between the variables. With the establishment of the relationship, the researchers moved to use of inferential statistics.

RESULTS

Three Hundred seventy-four (374) significantly disabled clients of the RSA closed in status 26 in fiscal year 1998 (e.g., cases closed by September 30, 1998) of the RSA are the observations. There are four predictor variables in the study, including highest grade completed, year last employed, and year of birth. As indicated in Table 1, the average weekly earnings is $322.49 with a standard deviation of $145.76. The means and standard deviations for the clients' birth year is 56.23 and 11.50, respectively; year employed: 94.40 and 3.99 respectively; and, highest grade completed: 11.66 and 2.62, respectively. See Table 2.

Figures 1, 2 and 3 are partial regression plots. They reveal the lineality of weekly earning of consumers in closed status 26 and the independent variables. Interpretations permit the researchers to reject the position of no relationship be-

TABLE 1. Descriptive Statistics

	Mean	Std. Deviation	N
WEEKLY EARNINGS AT CLOSURE	322.49	145.76	374
BIRTH YEAR	56.23	11.50	374
YEAR LAST EMPLOYED	94.40	3.99	374
HIGHEST GRADE COMPLETED	11.66	2.62	374

TABLE 2. Coefficients[a]

Model 1	Unstandardized Coefficients		Standardized Coefficients		
	B	Std. Error	Beta	t	Sig.
(Constant)	−106.406	166.899		−.638	.524
BIRTH YEAR	2.042	.601	.161	3.400	.001
YEAR LAST EMPLOYED	.776	1.734	.021	.448	.655
HIGHEST GRADE COMPLETED	20.648	2.646	.371	7.803	.000

a. Dependent Variable: WEEKLY EARNINGS AT CLOSURE

FIGURE 1. Partial Regression Plot: Weekly Earnings and Birth Year

Partial Regression Plot
Dependent Variable: WEEKLY EARNINGS AT CLOSURE

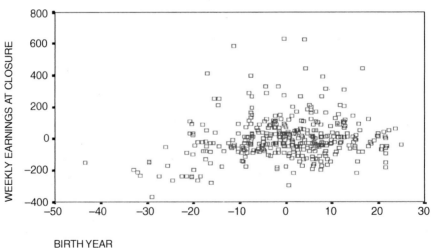

BIRTH YEAR

tween variables. In effect the researchers accept that there is a linear relationship between weekly earnings and birth year, highest grade completed and last year employed.

Regression analysis was used to determine which variables could be used to predict weekly earnings of significantly disabled consumers of the 1998 RSA closed in status 26. Variability in weekly earnings (17.2%) of the clients with

FIGURE 2. Partial Regression Plot: Weekly Earnings and Year Last Employed

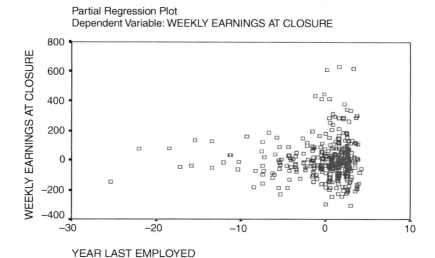

YEAR LAST EMPLOYED

FIGURE 3.

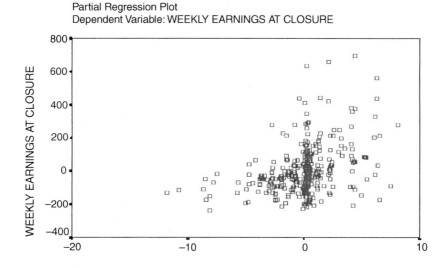

HIGHEST GRADE COMPLETED

significant disabilities can be predicted. Analysis of the dependent variable of earnings at closure, and predictors: the highest grade completed; birth year, and last year employed, produced an $F = 25.690$ with an $R2 = 0.172$.

CONCLUSION

This research provides the practitioner with an ability to connect formal policy and informal practices. The findings of this research can be used to provide a foundation for defining the predilection of successful employment outcomes for former welfare recipients (leavers). It posits that in order for leavers to move to a truly empowered state, they require not only training but education. Our ethics preclude harmful experimentation on human subjects, therefore when one population has traversed the process which can provide the data concerning possible outcomes, it is necessary to extrapolate that information and use it.

Education and work experience (work experience as the inverse periods of unemployment) is significantly related to earning power. Weekly earnings are significantly related to level of education, age and time since clients with significant disabilities had worked prior to eventually obtaining employment. This study provides indices which lay the framework for understanding possible outcomes of a similar population. Finally, society's willingness, as well as ability, to provide employment for those with disability is an indice for employability of other consumers in a temporary state of nonengagement. Consumers are the human resources for a capitalist society. These resources when undereducated, under trained and underdeveloped are not utilized to the full potential. The study suggests intervention for persons with significant disabilities at an early period in their life cycle. The findings of this study suggest that the public vocational rehabilitation program may need to take another look at how success is measured as it relates to serving clients with significant disabilities. Given these findings, service providers are particularly cautioned to pay attention to the age, prior work experience and educational needs of these consumers. There is a need for more research in this area to identify additional variables that may explain level of earnings for persons with significant disabilities.

REFERENCES

Adams, M. (2001). Race, disability: A double minority, (www.Sunspot.net/balto.blind 24jul24.story)
Akabas, S.H. and Gates, L.B. (1997). Managing disability in the workplace: A role for social workers, 239-255.

Becker, G.S. (1964), *Human capital*. New York: National Bureau of Economic Research.

Belgrave, F.Z. and Walker, S. (1991). Predictors of employment outcome of Black persons with disabilities, *Rehabilitation Psychology*, *36*(2), 111-119.

Brauner, S. and Loprest, P. (1999). Where are they now? What states' studies of people who left welfare tell us. *Assessing the new federalism*, Series A, No. A-32. Washington, DC. Urban Institute.

Brookins, G.K. (1998). Human capital and the W.K. Kellogg foundation mission. *International Journal*, *10*(1), 1-3.

Coe, N.B., Acs, G., Lerman, R.I. and Watson, K. (1998). Does work pay? A summary of the work incentives under TANF. *Assessing the new federalism*, Series A, No. A-28. Washington, DC.: Urban Institute.

Data from the 1995 Current Population Survey obtained from the Census Bureau Web site at <www.census.gov/hhes/www/disabled/disablecps.htm>

Dunham, M.D., Holliday, G.A., Douget, R.M., Koller, J.R., Presberry, R., Wooderson, S. (1998). Vocational rehabilitation outcomes of African American adults with specific learning disabilities. *Journal of Rehabilitation*, *64*(3), 36-41.

GAO (1996). People with disabilities, *GAO/HEHS-96-126*. Washington, DC. GAO.

Gittleman, M. (July 1994). Earnings in the 1980's: An occupational perspective, *Monthly Labor Review*.

Kurzman, P.A. and Akabas, S.H. (1993). *Work and well-being*. Washington, DC. NASW Press.

Lerman, R.I., Loprest, P. and Ratcliffe, C. (1999). How well can urban labor markets absorb welfare recipients? *Assessing the new federalism*, Series A, No. A-33. Washington, DC. Urban Institute.

Proctor, E.K. and Stiffman, A.R. (1998). Background of services and treatment research, 259-286, in William, J.B.W. and Ell, K. (Editors). *Advances in mental health research: Implications for practice*. Washington, DC. NASW Press.

Williamson, C. (1998). Social work practice with people with disabilities, p. 375-397 in Morales, A.T. And Sheafor, B.W. *Social work: A profession of many faces*. Boston: Allyn and Bacon.

Wright, B.A. (1968). *Physical disability–a psychological approach*. New York: Harper & Row.

Zedlewski, S.R., Holcomb, P.A. and Duke, A.E. (1998). Cash assistance in transition: The story of 13 states. *Assessing the new federalism*, Occasional paper number 16. Washington, DC. Urban Institute.

Foster Care Children with Disabilities

Jacqueline Marie Smith, PhD

SUMMARY. Each year the number of children who enter the foster care system grows because the number of children who are vulnerable to abuse, neglect and/or poverty grows. Children with disabilities are a particularly vulnerable subset of this already vulnerable population. What are the implications of conceptual and methodological issues in theories of disability for estimates of children with disabilities in foster care? To what extent do children in the foster care system have disabilities? What are implications of existing health care coverage strategies (Medicaid, managed care, etc.) for the health and well-being of foster care children with disabilities? Conceptual and operational definitions of disability are reviewed. Descriptive statistics based on a secondary analysis of 1998 administrative AFCARS data are used to summarize the extent of disabilities. In addition, existing empirical studies and public policies on national and state health care insurance strategies are analyzed. *[Article copies available for a fee from The Haworth Document Delivery Service: 1-800-HAWORTH. E-mail address: <docdelivery@haworthpress.com> Website: <http://www.HaworthPress.com> © 2002 by The Haworth Press, Inc. All rights reserved.]*

KEYWORDS. Foster care, disability, childhood disability

INTRODUCTION

Since the mid-nineties, there have been considerable changes in the policies and the service delivery structure for health care and social assistance pro-

Jacqueline Marie Smith is affiliated with the School of Social Work, Howard University.

[Haworth co-indexing entry note]: "Foster Care Children with Disabilities." Smith, Jacqueline Marie. Co-published simultaneously in *Journal of Health & Social Policy* (The Haworth Press, Inc.) Vol. 16, No. 1/2, 2002, pp. 81-92; and: *Disability and the Black Community* (ed: Sheila D. Miller) The Haworth Press, Inc., 2002, pp. 81-92. Single or multiple copies of this article are available for a fee from The Haworth Document Delivery Service [1-800-HAWORTH, 9:00 a.m. - 5:00 p.m. (EST). E-mail address: docdelivery@haworthpress.com].

grams. For more than 30 years, most federal income assistance for children came from the AFDC program. Most recently, the federal government has increasingly shifted the responsibility for children and families back to state governments by formulating new legislative policies and creating new programs. This "devolution" of federal responsibility is reflected in the passage of the Personal Responsibility and Work Opportunity Act of 1996 [P.L. 104-193], the creation of the Temporary Assistance for Needy Families (TANF) program, changes in eligibility requirements for Supplemental Security Income (Sullivan v. Zebley, 1990), the enactment of Title XXI of the Social Security Act [P. L. 105-33], and the establishment in 1997 of the State Children's Health Insurance Program.

Significant changes have also occurred in health care because of technological innovations. Increasingly, scientists have identified chemical compounds that can control behaviors derived from diseases like epilepsy, diabetes, congestive heart failure and asthma (Baker, 1994). Improved screening and medicines can now also prevent defects that occur at birth. Developments in assistive technology that include power wheelchairs, sonic and vision enhancement guides and nerve cell stimulators have removed barriers to functioning. For example, persons with spinal cord injuries who are fitted with electronic stimulators are able to return to the coordinated movements of walking because muscles contract from successive bursts of low-level controlled electrical stimulation (Smart, 2001:40; Scherer, 1993). These pharmological and engineering innovations have shifted the quality of life for children with functional and developmental limitations.

Structural or organizational shifts in the service delivery system of health care providers have also occurred (Simms et al., 1999). Health care providers have increasingly shifted from solo to group practices known as health maintenance organizations. The group practices contract with patients and organizations relatively elaborate plans for the delivery of health care services. The plans manage the delivery of service by contractually arranging and defining the process of diagnosis and treatment so that the cost of service delivery is constrained, capitated, and profitable (Fox et al., 1997). Thus, to some extent, the trend toward managed care plans represents a shift in the control of doctor-patient relationships from individual practitioners to group or corporate entities.

When change in society occurs quickly, and the changes radically reorder resources, social roles and responsibilities, social scientists tend to label it revolutionary (Tilly, 1993). Indeed, there is almost a "crowd" of scholars (e.g., Marx, Tilly, De Tocqueville) who examine populations and subgroupings in an effort to understand the benefits of social change and lessen its trauma. When change occurs less quickly, and/or there are mere institutional "shifts," rather than inversions of resources, roles and responsibilities, fewer scholars describe, explain and predict the impact of "reform" on population subgroups.

To some extent, this appears to have occurred in the area of foster care population with disabilities. Children in foster care are a subgroup in the population of children in the United States. Their numbers have grown over time. In 1965, there were approximately 300,000 children in foster care. By 1998, there were an estimated 568,000 children in care (Green Book, 2000). Foster care children with disabilities are a subgrouping of this subgroup. Furthermore, it seems likely that the cumulative effects of the most recent changes in the policy and social service delivery environment have been increased numbers of children entering out-of-home care because of poverty and significantly compromised health (Simms et al., 1999:169). Yet, the available literature on prevalence of children with disabilities in foster care (Sullivan, 2000), and the organization, delivery and financing of social and health care services for children with disabilities (Fox et al., 1997; GAO, 1996; American Academy of Pediatrics, 1998) or foster care children with disabilities is relatively scarce.

It could be reasonably argued that these technological and health care delivery changes (i.e., managed care) are particularly likely to affect the prevention, management and quality of life of foster care children with disabilities. In the past the Child Welfare League has asserted that " . . . (A)s a society we have failed to meet the health needs of many of the children in out-of-home care (CWLA, 1988:1)." What are we able to say about the children in foster care who have disabilities? Within this context, this study will: (a) identify and discuss the issues attached to the conceptualization and measurement of disability; (b) describe the prevalence or extent of disability in the foster care, and (c) discuss the implications of changes in the delivery of health care services (i.e., managed care) for prevention and management of chronic diseases for foster care children.

CONCEPTS OF DISABILITY

The concept of disability has been defined by legislators, administrators and researchers. Westbrook et al. (1998) have observed that at the federal level alone there are more than 40 different definitions of disability used primarily for programmatic purposes, planning and system development or research. The Social Security Disability Insurance Program defined disability as " . . . the inability to engage in substantial gainful activity by reason of any determinable physical or mental impairment that can be expected to result in death or to last for a continuous period of not less than twelve months (Disability Advisory Council, 1988:9)." The Individuals with Disabilities Education Act

(1990) defines children with disabilities as having any of the following types of disabilities: autism, deaf-blindness, hearing impairments (including deafness), mental retardation, multiple disabilities, orthopedic impairments, other health impairments, serious emotional disturbance, specific learning disabilities, speech or language impairments, traumatic brain injury, and visual impairments (including blindness). The World Health Organization (1980) in the International Classification of Impairment, Disabilities and Handicaps, defined disability as a health experience resulting from an impaired ability to perform an activity in a manner or within a range considered "normal." Social scientists also have a variety of definitions. LaPlante, for example, writes that a disability is ". . . a limitation–caused by one or more chronic physical or mental health conditions–in performing activities that people of a particular age are generally expected to be able to perform (LaPlante, 1991:34)." Smart (1998:45), on the other hand argues that the definition of disability should include "(1) the presence of a physical, intellectual, cognitive, or psychiatric condition; (2) (the presence of a) condition (that) impairs functioning; and (3) (that) the individual is subject to prejudice, discrimination, and reduced opportunity because of condition."

An examination of these definitions (La Plante, 1991; Smart, 2001; WHO, 1980; Westbrook, 1998) suggests that there are several commonalities. In most definitions, disability is a consequence of disease. In addition, the response to be the illness is assumed to be behavioral. The behavioral response tends to either physical/biological (sometimes defined as impairment), or social-psychological. Thus, an underlying assumption is that there are time ordered, directed, perhaps linear relationships between disease/illness and disability. Underlying the variety of definitions, however, there are also other common assumptions and propositions that structure and model the analytical representations of disability.

Writers argue that the assumptions, propositions and their applications in data collection, can be further grouped as theoretical models (Hahn, 1993; Smart, 1998). The dominant perspective, the medical model, is sometimes referred to as the categorical model (Perrin et al., 1993). The medical model focuses on the diagnosis of disease by medical experts. Causal explanations are thus limited to categories and often lack dimensionality and complexity. Furthermore, the cause of the disability resides within the individual, and the emphasis is on curing an individual's problem (Smart, 1998; Hahn, 1993).

Writers also suggest that some conceptualizations of disability reflect what is known as a functional model (Smart, 1998; Hahn, 1993). Programmatic and policy definitions of disability used to determine eligibility tend to fall within this school. In this context, the concept of disability captures an individual's restricted or reduced capacity to respond behaviorally to social role expectations. The severity and duration of an illness or pathological condition becomes the cause of an individual's restricted or reduced capacity to function in social roles like employee. Hahn (1993) argues that this perspective is largely focused on the economic domains of social life. Functional models of disability focus on measuring and representing performance of work activities and the activities of daily living. The WHO and Social Security program definitions described in earlier paragraphs of this narrative are examples of the functional model.

Critics and those interested in childhood disabilities have found these definitions and models of disability problematic for a variety of reasons (Simeonsson et al., 2000; Stein et al., 1997; Aron et al., 1996; Stein & Jessup, 1989). Such models of disability primarily address adult functioning. "As problems of learning constitute a major, if not the most important, manifestation of disabling conditions having congenital and developmental etiologies, lack of coverage of this and related domains constitutes a serious limitation (Simeonsson et al., 2000: 116)."

Furthermore, functional models (e.g., the International Classification of Impairments, Disabilities and Handicaps, [ICIDH] model) do not have a life span perspective. Thus, scant attention is paid to developmental issues in the areas of learning functioning at school, interacting with family or even functioning in family roles (Simeonsson et al., 2000). Overall, the medical and functional models neglect interaction with the environment.

Somewhat recently, writers have posited an environmental model (Smart, 2001). The environmental model tends to treat disability as a behavioral response to the social and physical environment. Disability, within this context, requires an interactive relationship with the environment. While the functional model primarily emphasizes the capacity for responses to social roles, the relationship between the social actor and the group is largely one-way.

In the environmental model, the experience of disability is treated as an interaction that is two-way rather than one-way (Brown, 1991). Internal and external environments are open rather than closed systems. The person who experiences disability can act in a manner to compensate and/or accommodate the environment, or the environment can respond to the functional capacity of individuals in such a way as to accommodate level of functioning. Writers like Hahn (1993) focus on the sociopolitical environment and its organization. He argues that the experience of disability should be recast as minority-majority group relationships in order to capture the dynamics of prejudice and discrimination. The definition of disability used in the Americans with Disabilities Act (ADA; P.L. 101-336) is illustrative of the environmental model. In the ADA, disability includes limitations in functions, as well as conditions/illness for which functional role limitations are not present because of some form of compensation at the level of the person in the environment.

DISABILITIES IN CHILDHOOD

Childhood disabilities can occur at birth or manifest over time. The many definitions of childhood disability reflect the social attitudes found in public policy, the prevailing theories of researchers at a particular time, as well as the general social period (Merrick, 2000). Definitions of disability experience for children share similarities with the general definitions of disability. Childhood disabilities are sometimes conceptualized as types or categories of diseases (Gortmaker & Sappenfield, 1984; Weiland et al., 1992). Childhood disabilities are also conceptualized as functional limitations. For example, Newacheck and Halfon (1998) define disability as a long-term reduction in the ability to conduct social role activities, such as school or play, because of a chronic physical or mental condition. This definition, then, tends to emphasize the functional capacity of children with chronic conditions to carry out expectations about social roles. Children's roles focus on the work of childhood because they do not have employment roles. Learning at school is a social work role for children. Similarly, play is an important work role for children because play is critical to social development.

MEASUREMENT OF DISABILITY IN CHILDHOOD

Researchers tend to:

1. use a checklist of chronic conditions;
2. a series of questions on self-care activities and/or
3. a series of questions on learning and play activities (Haber, 1991).

Data on children is generally collected from parent reports, school and medical records, and administrative records found in health care settings, rather than the self-reports of children.

The exclusive use of condition checklists seems likely to result in uneven coverage (i.e., underreporting) because of the rarity of some chronic conditions in childhood. Measures also may tend to over or underestimate disability because question content is not matched with the data source's knowledge. Some activity limitations may be more likely to manifest in the home setting, while others may be more likely to be revealed at school or on the playground. If a single, exclusive data source is used as a measure of prevalence, the measure may lack accuracy. Furthermore, the consistency of estimates may vary widely. Westbrook et al. (1998) found that using three different definitional components of disability yielded very different estimates of the disability.

The reliability of measures, however, is not the only methodological concern in measures of disability for children. The validity of measures also is of some concern because of the misspecification of causal models. Some models and definitions conceptualize disability as uni- rather than multidimensional. However, definitions that rely primarily on checklists of chronic conditions have little explanatory power.

The validity of measures in the context of existing theoretical models also requires some scrutiny. Data gathering and analysis of childhood disabilities are focused on the description of epidemiological rates rather than the causality of the disabling experience. The simplicity of the unidimensional concepts and linear, closed system relationships of the medical and functional models may lack the analytical power to generate rich, causal models of the experience of disability. In addition, model misspecification may provide poor quality data for the many persons who participate at some level in the experience of disability (person with the restriction, rehabilitation workers, social workers, therapists, etc.). Furthermore, validation studies of racial/ethnic differences need to be conducted (Newacheck et al., 1993).

PREVALENCE OF DISABILITY AMONG CHILDREN

When disability is measured by level of difficulty in performing everyday self-care activities like walking, eating, and activities associated with school performance like understanding school work, etc., a little more than 12% of children age 5-17 have difficulty in carrying out such tasks (National Institute of Child Health & Human Development, 2001). One tenth of all children with disabilities were unable to conduct their major school or play activities (Newacheck & Halfon, 1998:612). About 23% of those with disabling chronic conditions, were unable to attend school on a long-term basis (Newacheck and Halfon, 1998:613). Newacheck and Halfon (1998:614) estimated that five million hospital days could be attributed to childhood disability.

The extent of childhood disability varies by age and population subgroups. Boys are more likely than girls to have limitations of learning, communicating, mobility and self-care. Children who have limitations in learning, communicating, mobility or self-care tend to have a high use of the health care system. Westbrook et al. (1998) found that higher income children had more frequent reports of functional limitations than children from impoverished households did. Older children, and those from single parent households, also had higher rates of disability (Newacheck & Halfon, 1998).

CHILDREN IN FOSTER CARE WITH DISABILITIES

To what extent do children in the foster care system have disabilities? Data from the Adoption and Foster Care Analysis and Reporting System (AFCARS) were used to answer this question. The AFCARS data provides case level data for children served by the foster care system. The nature of AFCARS data does not permit multidimensional operational definitions of disability which are multidimensional and assume interaction with the environment. The content of questions asked in the original data collection focused exclusively on clinical diagnosed physical or psychological conditions. The content of the response to the original questions also did not provide information of functional limitations of performance, or the severity, duration and onset of the disabilities diagnosed by professionals. Thus, data present in this report can at best be regarded as gross indicators of the incidence of disability in the foster care population.

Children in care were more likely to be male (57%), white (43%) or African American (41%). Most children (48%) were over the age of 12. About 25% were age 7-11. Children were removed from their biological parents because of neglect (49%), physical abuse (16%) and sexual abuse (7%).

In 1998, there were 571,353 children under the age of 21 in the foster care system. AFCARS data show that no clinical assessment was conducted by a qualified professional for about 20% of the children who came into the system that year. Although clinical assessments determined that most children did not have disabilities, about 14% did. About .8% had visual or hearing impairments that might significantly affect educational performance or development. Two percent of children under age 21 had significantly below average general cognitive and motor functioning that could be labeled as mental retardation. A little more than 1% of children had physical conditions (e.g., cerebral palsy, spina bifida, multiple sclerosis, orthopedic impairments, etc.). Eight percent of children in foster care had psychological conditions that matched diagnosed mental disorders listed in the Diagnostic and Statistical Manual of Mental Disorders (DSM III-Third Edition). In addition to those with the conditions just described, almost 5% of the population under age 21 had other conditions (e.g., AIDS, HIV positive status, etc.) which required special care.

Some type or categories of disabilities varied by race. While there were slight or minimal racial/ethnic differences in the proportion of children diagnosed with visual or motor disabilities, there were larger differences between groups in mental retardation and mental disorders. Relatively smaller proportions of Asian Americans, Native Americans and persons of Hispanic origin were diagnosed with mental retardation and emotional disorders. More specifically, the proportion of Whites and African Americans with mental retardation was almost twice the proportion of Native Americans and Asian Americans. On the other hand, the proportions of White (11%), Native American (9%) and African American (7%) children in foster care with diagnosed mental disorders were greater than the proportions of Asian Americans with diagnosed mental disorders (5%).

Disabilities also varied with the age of children. When the ages of children were grouped into four categories: 0-3 years (infants and toddlers); 4-6 years (preschool); 7-12 (latency); and 13-21 (teenagers and young adults), there were minimal differences between age groups in visual hearing and motor disabilities. Greater proportions of older children were classified as mentally retarded. Greater proportions of children age 7-12 (2%) and age 13-21 (3%) were more often diagnosed as mentally retarded than infants and toddlers (.8%) and preschoolers (1%). Older children were also more frequently diagnosed with emotional disorders. More specifically, the proportions of children age 7-12 (7%) and 13-21 (13%) diagnosed with emotional disorders were greater than the proportions of children age 0-3 (.6%) and 4-6 years old (3%).

While it is not feasible to directly compare the incidence of disability of children in out-of-home placements with children in the general population because of differences in estimation technologies, it is reasonable to assume that the statistics cited here indicate substantial need for health and social services. Children in foster care have disproportionately high rates of physical, development and mental health needs (American Pediatric Association, 2000). Furthermore, children in foster care often have unmet medical and mental health needs (American Pediatric Association, 2000). Indeed, findings from the analysis presented here indicate that about 20% of children have received no assessment by a qualified professional.

Foster care children with health care needs are increasingly likely to have to negotiate the managed care environment. As the cost of Medicaid services exploded, states began turning to managed care. At the end of 1996, more than three quarters of States were serving Medicaid children through fully capitated plans, either on a statewide basis or in limited geographic areas (Fox et al., 1997: 26). "Although States were proceeding cautiously with managed care enrollment of foster care children and SSI children, they were rapidly AFDC and AFDC-related children with little attention to the special service requirements of those with disabilities" (Fox et al., 1997: 33).

However, the child with disabilities in the managed care environment is very different from the adults with disabilities. Children are different in that:

1. the dynamics of development affect needs and alter outcome;
2. childhood disabilities are often rare and infrequent conditions, and
3. children are dependent on their family's health and socioeconomic status (American Academy of Pediatrics, 1998).

In addition, children with rare disorders often experience multiple conditions requiring multiple interventions.

To enhance the quality of the degree of access of foster care children with disabilities, states might provide several incentives to managed care organizations. States might provide incentives to these organizations to develop clear standards of care and clinical guidelines for children with rare conditions. In addition, states should provide incentives for MCOs to integrate primary and specialty care that is needed by children who have multiple conditions.

AUTHOR'S NOTE

The data in this publication were made available by the National Data Archive on Child Abuse and Neglect, Cornell University, Ithaca NY, and have been used by permission. Data from *Adoption and Foster Care Analysis and Reporting System (AFCARS), 1998* were originally collected by the Children's Bureau, Administration on Children's. Funding was provided by the Children's Bureau, Administration on Children, Youth and Families, Administration for Children and Families, U.S. Department of Health and Human Services. Neither the collector of the original data, the funder, the Archive, Cornell University, or its agents or employees bear any responsibility for the analyses or interpretations presented here.

REFERENCES

American Academy of Pediatrics (1998, September). Managed care and children with special health care needs: A subject review. *Pediatrics, 102*(3).

American Academy on Pediatrics–Committee on Early Childhood, D.C. (2000, November). Developmental issues for young children in foster care. *Pediatrics, 106*(5).

Baker, D. W. (1994, November 2). Management of heart failure. Pharmacologic treatment. *Journal of the American Medical Association, 272*(17), 1361-1366.

Brown, S. C. (1991). Conceptualizing and defining disability. In S. Thompson-Hoffman & I. Storck (Eds.), *Disability in the United States: Portrait from national data.* New York, NY: Springer Publishing.

Child Welfare League of America (1988). *Standards for health care services for children in out-of-home care.* Washington, DC. Author.

Committee on Ways and Means. U. S. House of Representatives. (2000). *2000 Green book.* Washington, DC: U. S. Government Printing Office.

Disability Advisory Council (1988). Report of the Disability Advisory Council. Washington, DC: U. S. Department of Health and Human Services, Social Security Administration (1-78).

Fox, H. B., Margaret A, & Almeida, R. A. (1997, Summer). Medicaid managed care policies affecting children with disabilities: 1995 and 1996. *Health Care Financing Review, 18*(4).

Fox, P. D., & Fama, T. (1996). *Managed care and chronic illness* (P. D. Fox & T. Fama, Eds.). Gaithersburg, MD: Aspen Publishers.

Gortmaker, S. L., & Sappenfeld, W. (1984). Chronic childhood disorders: Prevalence and impact. *Pediatric Clinic North America, 31*.

Haber, Lawrence (1991). Operating definitions of disability: Survey and administrative measures. In S. Thompson-Hoffman & I. F. Storck (Eds.), *Disability in the United States: Portrait from national data*. New York, NY: Springer Publishing Company.

Hahn, H. (1993). Political implications of disability definitions and data. *Journal of Disability Policy Studies, 4*(2).

Horwitz, S. M., Owens, P., & Simms, M. D. (2000, July). Specialized assessments for children in foster care. *Pediatrics, 106*(1).

Individuals with Disabilities Education Act (1990). (Vol. 94-142) (Education of the Handicapped Act; Amended by P. L. 99-457).

LaPlante, M. (1991). Medical conditions associated with disability. In *Disability in the United States: Portrait from national data*. New York, NY: Springer Publishing Company.

LaPlante, M. P., & Carlson, D. (1996, August). Disability in the United States; prevalence and causes, 1992 [http://dsc.ucsf.edu/UCFS/pub.taf?_function=search&recid=65&grow=1] (Vol. Report 7) (06/09/01).

Merrick, J. (2000, April-September). Prevalence of disability in adolescence. *International Journal of Adolescent Medicine & Health, 12*(2-3).

Meyers, M., Lukemeyer, A., & Smeeding, T. (1998, June). The Cost of caring: Childhood disability and poor families. *Social Service Review*.

National Institute of Child Health & Human Development (2001, July). Federal interagency forum on child and family statistics [http://156.40.88.3/new/releases/CHIBAC1.htm] (July 24, 2001).

Newacheck, P. W., & Halfon, N. (1998, April). Prevalence and impact of disabling chronic conditions in childhood. *American Journal of Public Health, 88*(4).

Newacheck, P. W., Stoddard, J. J., & McManus, M. (1993, May). Ethnocultural variations in the prevalence and impact of childhood chronic conditions. *Pediatrics, 91*(5) (supplement).

Perrin, E., Newacheck, P., Pless, B., Drotar, D., Gortmaker, S. I., Leventhal, J., Perrin, J., Stein, R. E. K., Walker, D. K., & Weitzman, M. (1993, April). Issues involved in the definition and classification of chronic health conditions. *Pediatrics, 91*(4).

Perrin, J. M., & Stein, R., E. K. (1991, November). Reinterpreting disability: Changes in Supplemental Security Income for children. *Pediatrics, 88*(5).

Reisine, S., & Fifield, J. (1992). Expanding the definition of disability: Implications for planning, policy, and research. *The Milbank Quarterly, 70*(3).

Scherer, M. J. (1993). *Living in the state of stuck: How technology impacts the lives of people with disabilities*. Cambridge, MA: Brookline.

Simeonsson, R. J., Lollar, D., Hollowell, J., & Adams, M. (2000, February). Revision of the international classification of impairments, disabilities, and handicaps developmental issues. *Journal of Clinical Epidemiology, 53*(4).

Simms, M. D., Freundlich, M., Battistelli, & Kaufman, N. D. (1999, January/February). Delivering health and mental health care services to children in family foster care after welfare and health care reform. *Child Welfare, LXXVIII*(1).

Smart, J. (2001). *Disability, society and the individual.* Gaithersburg, MD: Aspen Publishers.

Stein, E. K. R., Westbrook, L. E., & Bauman, L. J. (1997, April). The Questionnaire for identifying children with chronic conditions: A measure based on a noncategorical approach. *Pediatrics, 99*(4).

Stein, R. E., & Jessup, D. J. (1992). A noncategorical approach to chronic childhood illness. *Public Health Reports, 37*(4).

Tilly, C. (1993). *European revolutions, 1492-1992.* Cambridge, MA: Blackwell.

United States General Accounting Office (1996). *Health insurance for children. State and private programs create new strategies to insure children.* Washington, DC (56).

Weiland, S., Pless, I. B., & Roghmann, K. J. (1992). Chronic illness and mental health problems in pediatric practice: Results from a survey of primary care providers. *Pediatrics, 89.*

Westbrook, L., Silver, E. J., & Stein, R. E. K. (1998). Implications for estimates of disability in children: A comparison of definitional components. *Pediatrics, 101*(June).

World Health Organization (1980). *International classification of impairments, disabilities, and handicaps.* Geneva: Author.

World Health Organization (1999). ICIDH2-B2 draft [http://www.who.chi/icidh] (07-13-01).

Public Housing Accommodations for Individuals with Disabilities

Samuel B. Little, PhD, LCSW-C

SUMMARY. The federal Housing Act of 1962 as amended and the subsequent laws of accommodations insure that all groups within American society, including those with disabilities, have access to housing opportunities. In spite of the clear provisions of various laws of accommodations enacted after 1962, it is questionable whether disabled individuals are adequately served by resident programs operated by Public Housing Agencies (PHAs) because rates of poverty, unemployment, domestic violence, and suicide are much higher among people with disabilities than in the nondisabled population. There are approximately 5 million residents living in 2.5 public housing units nationwide. New York, Puerto Rico, Chicago, Philadelphia and Baltimore have the five largest PHAs in the country. In combination, they rent 320,000 of the 1,300,495 inventory of rental properties owned by the country's 3,400 PHAs. Elderly and disabled residents without children account for 43% of all public housing families in the country. *[Article copies available for a fee from The Haworth Document Delivery Service: 1-800-HAWORTH. E-mail address: <docdelivery@haworthpress.com> Website: <http://www.HaworthPress.com> © 2002 by The Haworth Press, Inc. All rights reserved.]*

Samuel B. Little is Associate Deputy Director, Housing Authority of Baltimore City.

[Haworth co-indexing entry note]: "Public Housing Accommodations for Individuals with Disabilities." Little, Samuel B. Co-published simultaneously in *Journal of Health & Social Policy* (The Haworth Press, Inc.) Vol. 16, No. 1/2, 2002, pp. 93-107; and: *Disability and the Black Community* (ed: Sheila D. Miller) The Haworth Press, Inc., 2002, pp. 93-107. Single or multiple copies of this article are available for a fee from The Haworth Document Delivery Service [1-800-HAWORTH, 9:00 a.m. - 5:00 p.m. (EST). E-mail address: docdelivery@haworthpress.com].

KEYWORDS. Public Housing Authority (PHA), resident programs, reasonable accommodations, Section 504, workforce preparation resident councils, Jobs Plus demonstrations, computer technology Personal Responsibility and Work Opportunity Reconciliation Act of 1996 (PRWORA)

Data collected by the National Association of Housing and Redevelopment Officials (NAHRO) show that 24% of the resident population in public housing is comprised of disabled non-elderly and 30% of disabled elderly residents. From the date it is clear that disabled individuals occupy a sizable proportion of housing units in this country. However, it is questionable whether disabled residents have similar access to many of the PHA operated resident programs that provide supportive services to non-elderly residents.

This article discusses public housing accommodations for residents with disabilities. Over the years, many PHAs have administered social service programs providing family counseling, work force development activities, child and adult care services, recreation, substance abuse prevention, health screening, housing assistance, meal service and other initiatives that promote self-sufficiency of families. The basic objective of these programs has been to enhance the lives of housing residents, but participation rates by disabled individuals have been relatively small when compared to the number of disabled families living in public housing that might need supportive services.

There is concern that the recent shift by the Bush administration to transfer responsibility for social service programs from PHAs to faith-based organizations may cause many disabled persons to fall through the cracks of the service system. Therefore, the present challenge for PHAs is to widen, rather than reduce, options for disabled residents to participate in social service programs, enforce direct and open recruitment of disabled persons in job training or other employment strategies, and tailor special events to individual capabilities.

The promise of affordable, safe and decent housing may be a limited reality rather than a guarantee for too many disabled individuals unless "reasonable accommodation" policies are combined with "reasonable expectation" policies enacted by PHAs. The two must go hand-in-hand if disabled persons living in public housing developments and Section 8 properties are to be helped to maintain an acceptable level of independence and autonomy.

The promise of affordable, safe and decent housing is a basic guarantee of the federal Housing Act of 1962 as amended. Passed in response to a pressing need to ensure that all groups within American society, including those with disabilities, have access to housing opportunities, the importance of the Housing Act was echoed further by the subsequent passage of the Architectural Barriers Act of 1968, Rehabilitation Act of 1973, Public Law 94-42 (later renamed the Individuals with Disabilities Education Act of 1975 or IDEA), Fair Housing Act of 1988, and Americans with Disabilities Act of 1990 (ADA). Many individuals locked outside mainstream society, from impoverished and disenfranchised communities to those with a physical or mental impairment, believe these laws of accommodation guarantee their access to education, employment, and housing in the public and private domain regardless of ethnicity, age, income, physical condition, or personal circumstance that may entangle their lives.

Each of these laws has clearly stated purposes and provisions. Nonetheless, housing professionals and policy analysts debate whether individuals with disabilities are adequately served today because rates of poverty, unemployment, underemployment and suicide are much higher among disabled persons as compared to the nondisabled population (Haber, 1990). There is ample evidence in the literature to substantiate that many people with disabilities tend to "fall through the cracks" of the service system and do not have sufficient accommodations such as disability benefits (Timmons, 2000), accessible transportation and parking, personal care providers (Gilmore and Butterworth, 2000), subsidized and affordable housing (Newman, 1999), assistance with independent living, vocational rehabilitation (Murphy, 2001), work force development opportunities (Harrison, 1998), computer technology and the Internet (Kaye, 2000), or other services that promote self-sufficiency and independence.

Beyond bipartisan consensus about laws of accommodation that were to signal a new level of participation for Americans with a disability, there is a need to enhance the disability rights movement in this country if for no other reason than to amend conflicting attitudes held toward persons with disabilities. As reflected by Justice William Joseph Brennon, Jr., writing in a Supreme Court decision, "society's accumulated fears and myths about disabilities and diseases are as handicapping as are the physical limitations that flow from actual impairment" (School Board of Nassau County v. Arline, 107s. Ct. 1123, 1987). The concern intensifies when Brennon's perspective factors in the notion that disabled individuals living in public housing developments are likely to face circumstances that threaten their immediate well-being, are among those with the fewest resources, are frequently isolated from institutions designed to provide assistance, have incomes too low to purchase services at market price, and may be reluctant to seek services because of stigmatization and eligibility requirements.

Attitudes of members of society are as important as the various laws of accommodation. For this reason, housing professionals, politicians, advocacy organizations and other groups are compelled to focus attention on rectifying not only the misconceptions and mythical thinking about individuals with disabilities, but to adequately assist disabled families residing in public housing developments and other low-income communities. In these communities, the disabled person is likely to experience high rates of crime, domestic violence, substance abuse, drug trafficking, joblessness, deteriorating physical conditions, and other social problems that disenfranchise individuals and produce dysfunctional family status.

DEFINITION OF DISABILITY

There is no one standard definition of disability. However, with the passage of various laws of accommodation, use of an operational definition of disability becomes increasingly important in the emporium of human interactions if there is to occur a meaningful examination of the myriad of challenges confronting professionals who serve this population. Each of the laws cited previously adapted a similar definition of disability. Additionally, it is clear in the language in these laws that the phrase "individual with disabilities" has the same meaning as the term "individual with handicaps." Under 24 C.F.R 8.3 of ADA, for example, individuals with handicaps means "any person who has a physical or mental impairment that substantially limits one or more major life activities; has a record of such an impairment; or is regarded as having such impairment." Generally, major life activities refer to those activities a typical individual can perform with little or no difficulty such as walking, breathing, seeing, hearing, speaking and working.

Disabled individuals comprise a significant and growing population in the United States. Data gathered from the Survey of Income and Program Participation (SIPP) administered in 1997 by the U.S. Department of Commerce, estimate that 52.6 million people in the United States have some level of disability and 33.0 million of these individuals can be considered to have a severe disability. This represents 19.7% of the non-institutionalized civilians in the country. The data also show that the prevalence of disability by selected characteristics increases with age; varies by race, sex and definitions of disability status; reflects poverty status, educational attainment, and health conditions; is a factor determining whether an individual has insurance protection; and is associated with receiving welfare benefits and other forms of cash assistance.

In addition to these characteristics, data gathered from SIPP estimate that 15.0 million non-institutionalized residents in the country have an activity limitation; 14.3 million people are limited in the kind or amount of major activity they can perform; and 19.9 million persons are limited in activities other than major activity such as playing, attending school, working or keeping house, bathing, eating, dressing, performing household chores, shopping or doing necessary business. In combination, these statistics explain the growing number of disabled people requiring assistance in daily activities and the importance of collaborative efforts on their behalf between housing professionals and external service providers in the community.

ROLE OF PUBLIC HOUSING AGENCIES

The U. S. Housing Act of 1937, commonly known as the Wagner-Steagall Act, authorized the public housing program in this country. It was the first major federal program aimed at providing low-rent housing to low-income households. Today, the U.S. Department of Housing and Urban Development (HUD) administers Federal assistance to local Public Housing Agencies (PHAs) and redevelopment agencies. The primary purpose of these programs is to provide decent shelter for low-income residents at rents they can afford.

Based on 1998 data gathered by the Council on Large Public Housing Agencies (CLPHA), there are 3,400 PHAs nationwide. Additional data compiled by CLPHA estimate that PHAs and redevelopment agencies house more than 5 million individuals within their inventory of 2.5 million rental units.

New York, Puerto Rico, Chicago, Philadelphia, and Baltimore have the five largest PHAs in the country. Collectively, these public agencies rent more than 320,000 units out of 1,300,493 rental properties that comprise the inventory of CLPHA member agencies. Unmarried women with two or more children and the elderly rent the majority of these units. Each PHA maintains an average occupancy rate of 78% of the existing unit mix.

In Maryland, for example, the Housing Authority of Baltimore City (HABC) is the state's largest PHA and landlord. HABC houses 40,000 residents, administers more than 13,000 Section 8 certificates and manages 16,000 of the state's 24,204 pool of rental units. This picture is similar in a significant number of communities across the country in which the local PHA is also the area's biggest landlord.

Many PHAs are not only in a unique position to accommodate a large number of individuals with disabilities, they are expected to do so as a pivotal landlord in the public sector. PHAs also have reasonable accommodation policies and procedures to ensure participation by disabled persons in public housing programs and activities. HUD requires PHAs to accommodate individuals with disabilities by providing assessable features in the housing unit. Examples include Section 504 units (i.e., those assessable by wheelchair or equipped with hearing and vision apparatus), qualified interpreters, or telecommunications devices for the deaf person. Each housing development has a limited number of 504 units that are frequently not equal to the number of disabled individuals who may need special accommodations. Nonetheless, PHAs and re-development agencies have an obligation to ensure that their policies, practices and resident programs address the needs of disabled individuals by either providing or linking them with supportive services and work force development activities. These services are designed to maximize their potential to become stable, healthy, and productive members of the community, as well as to help them achieve self-sufficiency.

CHARACTERISTICS OF HOUSING RESIDENTS

Public housing is a valuable source of housing for the most vulnerable elderly and disabled populations in American society. According to the National Association of Housing and Redevelopment Officials (NAHRO), elderly and disabled households without children account for 43% of all public housing families in the country. This represents approximately 560,000 families residing in the 1.3 million rental units nationwide. However, 24% of the resident population is comprised of disabled non-elderly and 30% of disabled elderly tenants. These percentages do not include elderly and disabled households who also have dependent children.

In addition, NAHRO data confirm that most families live in public housing units less than 10 years, and 40% remain three years or less. But those who stay longer include low-income elderly and disabled residents who have no other source of housing. The average household monthly rent for public housing residents is $193.

Although there are no data to document the precise number of disabled residents who rely on mobility aids, it has been observed that at most PHAs around the country, disabled individuals use wheelchairs, canes or walkers. Many have difficulty performing functional activities such as speaking, lifting, seeing or hearing. Others have mental or emotional conditions that seriously interfere with everyday activities and receive federal benefits based on an inability to work.

Table 1 gives selected resident characteristics for the five largest PHAs in the country. At each housing agency, there are a sufficient number of disabled non-elderly and disabled elderly residents who may experience particular circumstances which restrict them to their developments. New York City and Chicago lead the country in terms of accommodating the largest number of non-elderly disabled residents. Chicago and Philadelphia serve the largest number of elderly disabled residents. Baltimore performs better than Puerto Rico that has four times the number of housing residents.

TABLE 1. Selected Characteristics of Public Housing Authorities

PHA	Estimated # of Tenants	Occupancy Rate	Av. Family Size	Disabled Non-Elderly Tenants (%)	Disabled Elderly Tenants (%)
New York City	392,696	90	2.4	24	30
Puerto Rico	177,260	97	3.2	9	11
Chicago	71,753	72	2.5	27	87
Philadelphia	45,483	71	2.5	16	61
Baltimore	40,411	78	2.1	19	25

Source: Picture of Subsidized Households, 1998

In this country, the majority of disabled residents are female heads of households who live with other family members who are frequently young children (Kaye, 2000). Medium income is approximately $26,400 annually. However, in Baltimore, the median income of disabled persons in public housing is under $10,000 annually. The average age of the disabled person is 38 years and 63 years for elderly residents. Both groups have less that a high school diploma. While the domain of disability cannot be identified for the four largest PHAs, census data show that disabled persons generally experience mental symptoms that seriously interfere with daily activities such as coping with stress, anxiety, concentrating, and getting along with others.

The results of a recent survey of 190 disabled residents at nine HABC developments have produced a profile of some of the distinguishing characteristics of disabled individuals. The developments were Douglass, Latrobe, Pleasant View Gardens, Cherry Hill, Gilmor, McCulloh, O'Donnell, Somerset and the Terraces. All are designated family developments, housing elderly and non-elderly families. Pleasant View Gardens and the Terraces were redeveloped during the past four years as part of the HOPE VI Revitalization and Demonstration Program.

Of the 30 disabled residents surveyed at Pleasant View Gardens, age ranged between 26 and 74 years. For the majority, the source of income was Supplemental Security Income (SSI) and all were unemployed at the time of the survey. Disability was the result of degenerative bone disease, substance abuse, congestive heart failure, hearing impairment, multiple sclerosis or being wheelchair bound. At the Latrobe development, 30 of the 50 residents surveyed were females, and the majority or 24 presently receive SSI as compared to much smaller numbers receiving Veterans Benefits (VA), Temporary Emergency Medical Health Assistance (TEMHA), and Old Age Survival Insurance (OASI). Five have no source of income and rely on family members for their livelihood. It should be noted that disabled residents have access to a range of resident services including case management, transportation, computer classes and substance abuse treatment services. Documentation also showed that the residents surveyed have difficulty organizing daily living tasks and managing medication intake. They also were lacking in sufficient support from family members, faced employment discrimination, and were frequently isolated from other sources of support.

HUD requires PHAs to provide "reasonable accommodations" to residents with disabilities (48 FR 00638, republished at 48 FR 22470, May 13, 1983). As such, PHAs established a reasonable accommodation policy and procedures to comply with Section 504 of the Rehabilitation Act of 1973. The act prohibits discrimination on the basis of disability status and states that:

> No qualified individual with handicaps shall, solely on the basis of hand-icap be excluded from participation in, be denied the benefit of, or other-wise be subjected to discrimination under any program or activity that receives Federal financial assistance from the Department.

There are, for example, Section 504 dwelling units at all housing programs in the country. Reasonable accommodation activities under HABC's jurisdiction include, in addition to public housing, Section 8, rental partnership housing, and privatized HOPE VI communities. The reasonable accommodations policy of HABC is committed to ensuring all provisions of the Rehabilitation Act of 1973 and such accommodations, unless doing so would result in a fundamental alteration of the nature of the program, or an undue financial or administrative burden. In such cases, HABC will make another accommodation that would not result in a financial or administrative burden.

Table 2 shows a breakdown of HABC's Section 504 units by type of accommodations and bedroom size. Housing management officials confirm that the majority of requests filed by disabled HABC residents are for wheelchair accommodations. The real test is whether HABC is capable of providing reasonable accommodations to all individuals making such requests. According to the data that is consistent with this pattern shown in Table 2, the majority of the 504 units are rented to disabled residents who use an ambulatory aid such as a wheelchair, cane, crutches, or a walker.

In spite of laws of accommodations and the number of available housing units with appropriate accommodations for disabled residents, at times the commitment of the PHA to assist disabled residents is disputed by disabled persons, immediate family members, or advocacy groups such as the Maryland Disability Law Center (MDLC). During the past year, MDLC profusely argued at the annual meeting to present HABC's Five-Year Plan that disabled

TABLE 2. Type of Accommodations by Bedroom Size

	0 BR	1 BR	2 BR	3 BR	4 BR	5 BR	6 BR	TOTAL
Wheelchair	411	265	97	28	3	3	1	438
Hearing/Vision	33	57	36	19	1	1	0	147
Miscellaneous	114	216	46	18	11	0	0	405
Total	188	538	179	65	15	4	1	990

Source: Housing Authority of Baltimore City, 2001

housing residents are frequent victims of widespread situational discrimination, are denied access to essential supportive services, and do not receive the accommodations mandated by Federal law.

Officers and members of Resident Councils (sometimes called tenant associations) also have expressed the view that government leaders and public housing administrators show little interest in the welfare of disabled families and give only lip service to assist them to improve their overall situation. Other complaints from disabled housing residents point out inhumane building conditions, inadequate agency funding for supportive services, insufficient security services, questionable leasing procedures, and inequities in housing management practices. In combination, the different perspectives suggest a need to improve areas of internal program coordination and strengthen the existing linkages with external agencies that promote self-sufficiency and independence for disabled residents.

The sources of income for the majority of public housing residents are Temporary Assistance for Needy Families (TANF), SS, SSI, disability income or other forms of cash assistance. Baltimore mirrors the national trend in terms of sources of income. An analysis of data reported in the Multifamily Tenant Characteristics System maintained by the HUD shows that for the 24,204 public housing units in Maryland, for example, TANF, SS and SSI are the sources of income for 73% of residents as compared to 44% of residents occupying the inventory of 16,000 rental units in Baltimore City.

There is much to be done given the magnitude and scope of need of disabled residents. As PHAs have developed the HUD-required five-year plans that detail their focus for improving housing inventory, operations and resident services, they have an opportunity to upscale their commitment to disabled families. There is an increased need nationwide to serve physically and mentally disabled persons as well as those with chronic mental illnesses (CMI) and substance abuse histories. Based on HUD reports, only 25 of 41 PHAs have approved "designated housing" plans, giving them the green light to build housing to augment accommodations for residents with disabilities. Accommodations and supportive services are an important element for helping residents with disabilities.

RESIDENT SERVICES AND PROGRAMS

As the five largest PHAs in the country, New York City, Puerto Rico, Chicago, Philadelphia and Baltimore manage a diverse network of supportive services and economic development programs for the general resident population. These resident programs are usually located on-site at housing developments and provide family counseling, employment referrals, child and adult care services, recreation, substance abuse prevention, health screening, assisted housing, meal service, and other initiatives that promote self-sufficiency of families. The basic objective of these programs is to enhance the lives of participants and support their family unit overall.

Social analysts argue that the intent of resident programs is to be inclusive, serving all groups in need within the public housing community. At many PHAs, resident programs are designed to be "user friendly" and accommodate disabled residents, but it is frequently observed that participation rates in the basic self-sufficiency programs are small when compared to the total number of disabled persons living in public housing who would benefit from the programs. These programs include work force development strategies (job training and employment preparation activities), basic education and literacy services, recreation, and welfare-to-work. However, a two-fold dilemma faced by many PHAs is the growing number of disabled individuals seeking and obtaining public housing nationwide during an era of reduced federal funding for self-sufficiency programs, and a philosophical shift in responsibility for resident programs to faith-based organizations by the George Bush administration. Existing program resources are grossly insufficient to adequately serve disabled individuals who have limited options elsewhere in the marketplace. Frequently, the presence of on-site resident programs eliminates the need for disabled residents to travel outside the community for various supportive services. These are examples of some of the particular challenges that can confront PHAs elsewhere in the country.

Adults and Elderly Persons

Adult Medical Day Care, Elderly Service Coordination Program and Congregate Housing Service are among the familiar resident programs administered by many PHAs across the country. They target elderly and non-elderly disabled residents. In addition to providing services from therapists and physicians as deemed necessary, they provide meal service, transportation, light housekeeping, personal care and other basic services required to maintain residents in their homes and prevent institutionalization. In Baltimore, for example, two Adult Medical Day Care centers accommodate 80 residents. About half of the participants are disabled residents. At four other housing developments, the Elderly Service Coordination Program is administered, serving more than 5,225 units of services annually. In addition to meal service, the lives of disabled residents are enhanced further by providing them awareness training, immunization shots, attendance at concerts, talent shows, poetry recitals, senior companion services, and ethnic dinners.

Disabled residents also benefit from Psycho-Social Assessment and Treatment in City Housing (PATCH), a program intended to meet mental health needs of disabled residents by utilizing psychiatric nurses and psychiatrists to provide in-home assessment, treatment and referral services. Additionally, the Congregate Housing Service is available to residents at eight elderly housing developments. Collectively, these sites serve approximately 225 participants daily. Disabled residents comprise 60% of the participants of whom 10% are disabled persons under the age of 40.

Documentation in the case files of disabled residents sheds light on the problems disabled elderly residents experience, identifies gaps in the existing service delivery systems, and describes personal needs that arise on a regular basis. For example, issues of accessibility have been documented most often. All disabled residents are not presently assigned to a housing unit that is sufficiently equipped with handicap amenities such as grab bars, high toilets, lower sinks, cabinets with knobs or large handles, lower light switches, wide doors, no-slip floor covering, and hand-held shower fixtures. In some instances, the head of household has the disability and she or he is dependent on other family members due to the physical barriers in the home.

Several residents purchased their homes through the HOPE VI program, but have since become disabled and are faced with losing it because the disabled member must move to another unit that can only accommodate one person. Other disabled residents have expressed concern about living in developments that are excluded from the public transportation network and their inability to conduct activities of daily living such as shopping, banking, keeping appointments, or attending church and social events.

Issues of eligibility pose a set of unique problems as well. For example, medical transportation is not provided to non-medical assistance and Medicare disabled recipients. Resources for vision, dental, hearing apparatus, medical equipment, and wheelchairs are also excluded. Age requirements for certain services eliminate young disabled for personal care and other basic services.

Programs for Children and Youth

According to *Disabilities Sourcebook* (2000), the national statistics on disabilities indicate that 3.8 million or 5.5% of all families have children with disabilities. However, it is not always clear to what extent existing children and youth are effectively served as disabled housing residents nationwide. Nonetheless, at many PHAs, resident programs serving children and youth outnumber programs targeted to other age groups. For example, Head Start Centers, before-and-after child care programs, Boys and Girls Clubs, Police Athletic League Centers, 4-H Clubs and other organized recreational, educational and cultural enrichment activities are available to accommodate children and youth in public housing.

At licensed day care centers operated by HABC, for example, services are provided to children with physical and mental disabilities if they are able to function in the various centers without special assistance from staff. Currently, the number of disabled children served is less than 5% of the overall enrollment. These are children with a disfigurement as well as thrive infants or toddlers. External service vendors usually provide these residents supportive services and case management. Several youth participants are confined to wheelchairs, require ramp accessibility, and have visible handicaps. The Child Care Administration has established a special subsidy rate for children with disabilities enrolled in purchase of care programs.

Employment and Career Opportunities

Job opportunities in many cities are expanding each year in response to the healthy economy. Over half of the new jobs will be in highly skilled professional, technical and managerial occupations. In spite of economic good health, the President's Committee on Employment of People with Disabilities reported in 1996 that 70% of working people with disabilities are unemployed.

Out of 2,723 cases or housing residents enrolled in work force development programs, about 60 have documented disabilities. Two are in business or entrepreneurialship training. Local housing professionals express a major concern reported by employers about hiring people with disabilities: matching skills and needs, supervision and training, cost associated with safety and medical insurance premiums, legal liabilities and making the workplace accessible. Many of these are similar to those reported in the research conducted by Harrison (1998).

In addition to literacy and occupational skills training, an important work force development strategy is to bridge the digital divide among disabled persons who are less than half as likely as their non-disabled counterparts to own a computer. Computer technology and the Internet have a tremendous potential to broaden the career lives and increase the independence of people with disabilities. Computers can offer access to information, social interaction, cultural activities, employment options, and consumer products. Voice recognition, for example, can enable disabled residents with limited dexterity to write letters, manage their finances, or perform work-related tasks. In public housing communities, disabled individuals represent a rich pool of qualified workers that can enrich the changing marketplace.

Under the Personal Responsibility and Work Opportunity Reconciliation Act of 1996 (PRWORA), recipients of welfare are encouraged to improve their economic status by returning to or entering employment. Nonetheless, the emphasis on employment presents challenges to case managers in resident programs who are responsible for helping their disabled clients acquire the necessary skills and training to enter employment. Residents with disabilities offer an additional challenge to case managers who previously were not required to be familiar with disability-specific support, disability rights protection, and employment support.

At seven PHAs in the country (Seattle, Baltimore, St. Paul, Chattanooga, Los Angeles, Cleveland and Dayton), Jobs-Plus demonstrations are underway to test the merits of saturating a housing development with supportive services as not only an effective solution to ending welfare dependency and unemployment, but to assist housing residents to become self-sufficient at a housing development. The program operates under the auspices of Manpower Demonstration Research Corporation (MDRC), based in New York City. The program in Baltimore is located at Gilmor Homes, a family development with 225 families. Only three disabled families are assisted, yet 504 dwelling unit data show that 43 units or 7.6% of the units are targeted to individuals with disabilities. A limitation of the program may be its inability to recruit and serve adults with disabilities.

Since the passage of welfare reform legislation in 1997, an abundance of research has focused on public housing residents and other low-income individuals making the transition from welfare to work, leaving the nation's welfare rolls, or entering new careers in urban and rural growth markets. Social work researchers have not sufficiently examined issues related to housing accommodations for individuals and families with disabilities. It is reasonable to conclude that individuals with identified and suspected disabilities in public housing are often not effectively served because of geographic isolation from the agencies that target them for service, but equally because housing professionals lack training and expertise to respond to the complexities faced by such individuals. Additionally, at many PHAs, supportive services personnel are not linked with professionals in other disciplines to take advantage of advocacy, technical assistance, referral activity and other sources of help that could directly benefit disabled residents. However, it should be noted that state-level organizations that provide support and resources to individuals with disabilities are located in states with large public housing populations.

CONCLUSIONS

The promise of affordable, safe and decent housing may be a limited reality rather than a guarantee to many disabled individuals in public housing. For certain groups entangled by circumstances beyond their control, affordable housing has a dichotomous meaning that includes the physical unit and the supportive services necessary to maintain an acceptable level of independence and autonomy.

PHAs in central cities and small towns comprise an enormous network of housing opportunity for disabled individuals specifically, but to others disenfranchised or locked outside mainstream society. Increased attention needs to be placed on preventing disabled individuals in public housing from falling through the cracks of the service system. The national statistics on individuals with disabilities are significant and so are the numbers of disabled persons in public housing that are not participants in resident programs that were designed to enhance their quality of life.

As public landlords, PHAs must bridge the present gap in service opportunity created by strongly-held myths about disabled persons, sometimes policies and procedures imposed by Boards of Commissioners at the advice of housing experts, and frequently gross neglect or insensitivity on the part of those administering public housing programs in this country. Reasonable accommodations policies without reasonable expectations of the policies are counterproductive. The two must go hand-in-hand.

At many PHAs, there is a resident program infrastructure to address basic needs of elderly individuals. Programs for adults, children and youth, and those transitioning from welfare to work are not utilized to the fullest by disabled housing residents. The challenge for housing officials is to widen options for persons with disabilities within agency-run resident programs, enforce direct and open recruitment of housing residents in job training and employment strategies, and tailor special events to individual capabilities. These are among the necessary steps to bridge the opportunity gap in order to achieve the promises of various laws of accommodations enacted on behalf of disabled individuals.

REFERENCES

Abberly, P. (1989). Disability people: Normality and social work. In L. Burton (Eds.), *Disability and Dependency.* London: Falmer.

Daniels, N. (1997). Mental disability, equal opportunity, and the ADA. In R. Bonnie & J. McNahan (Eds.), *Mental Disorder, Work Disability and the Law.* Chicago: University of Chicago Press.

Fink, D. B. (2000). *Making a Place for Kids with Disabilities.* Connecticut: Praeger Publishers.

Franck, K. (1998). Assisted living in public housing: A case study of mixing frail elderly and younger persons with chronic mental illness and substance abuse histories. In D. P. Varady, P. F. E. Wolfgang, & Russell, F. (Eds.), *New Directions in Urban Public Housing* (pp. 61-84). New Jersey: Center for Urban Policy Research Press.

Gilmore, D. S. & Butterworth, J. (2000). Work status trends for people with mental retardation. *Research to Practice,* 4, 1-3.

Haber, L.D. (1990). Issues in the definition of disability and the use of disability survey data. In D. B. Levin, M. Zitter & L. Ingram (Eds.), *Disability Statistics: An Assessment* (pp. 35-51). Washington, DC: National Academy Press.

Harrison, O. (1998). Employing people with disabilities: Small business concerns and recommendations (pp. 21-27). *Research to Practice,* 5, 1-7.

Hopkins, K. (1991). Public attitudes toward people with disabilities. *Willing to Act (p. 7).* Washington, DC: National Organization on Disability.

Kaye, S. H. (2000). Disability and the digital divide (pp. 1-5). *Disability Statistics Center Abstract,* 22, 1-4.

Longmore, P. K. & Umansky, L. Eds. (2001). The New Disability History: American Perspectives (pp. 33-52). New York: New York University Press.

Matthews, D. D. Eds. (2000). In *Disabilities Sourcebook* (pp. 11-19, 35-60). Detroit: Frederick G. Ruffner, Jr., Publishers.

McNeil, J. (2001). Americans with disabilities. In *Current Population Reports.* U.S. Census Bureau, Economic and Statistics Administration.

Oliver, M. (1986). Social policy and disability: Some theoretical issues. *Disability, Handicap and Society.* 1, 5-18.

Schneider, J. W. (1988). Disability as moral experience: Epilepsy and self in routine relationships. *Journal of Social Issues,* 44, 63-78.

Silvers, A., Wasserman, D. & Mahowald, M. (1998). *Disability, Difference, Discrimination: Perspectives on Justice in Bioethics and Public Policy* (pp. 226-291). New York: Rowman and Littlefield Publishers.

Temelini, D. & Fesko, S. (1998). Disability organizations' perspective on the needs of youth with disabilities who are runaway or homeless. *Research in Practice,* 4, 31-42.

Timmons, J. C. & Drelinger, D. (2000). Time limits, exemption, and disclosure: TANF caseworkers and clients with disabilities. *Research in Practice,* 3, 41-48.

Addressing Students'
Social and Emotional Needs:
The Role of Mental Health Teams in Schools

Norris M. Haynes, PhD

SUMMARY. Children in today's society face many stresses from a variety of sources that have a major impact on thier psychosocial adjustment and academic performance in school. These stressful events and thier consequences on the quality of life and academic success are particularly significant among low-income and ethnic minority students in American society. Many schools have adopted strategies to help students who are impacted by stressful life events to deal affectively with their problems in an attempt to reduce school failure and school dropout rates among these students. Most notable among these strategies are school-based mental health programs including the establishment of school-based mental health teams which seek to proactively address individual student concerns while improving the general climate of schools. The evidence seems to support the claim that these school-based services have a positive impact on students' social and emotional well-being as well as on their academic achievements. However, with more careful monitoring and much more consistent support from administrators and policy mak-

---

Norris M. Haynes is Professor, Counseling and School Psychology Director, Center for Community and School Action Research (CCSAR), Southern Connecticut State University.

[Haworth co-indexing entry note]: "Addressing Students' Social and Emotional Needs: The Role of Mental Health Teams in Schools." Haynes, Norris M. Co-published simultaneously in *Journal of Health & Social Policy* (The Haworth Press, Inc.) Vol. 16, No. 1/2, 2002, pp. 109-123; and: *Disability and the Black Community* (ed: Sheila D. Miller) The Haworth Press, Inc., 2002, pp. 109-123. Single or multiple copies of this article are available for a fee from The Haworth Document Delivery Service [1-800-HAWORTH, 9:00 a.m. - 5:00 p.m. (EST). E-mail address: docdelivery@haworthpress.com].

10.1300/J045v16n01_10

ers, these school-based approaches can more fully realize their potential to enhance the quality of life and to positively impact the future of many poor and ethnic minority students. *[Article copies available for a fee from The Haworth Document Delivery Service: 1-800-HAWORTH. E-mail address: <docdelivery@haworthpress.com> Website: <http://www.HaworthPress.com> © 2002 by The Haworth Press, Inc. All rights reserved.]*

KEYWORDS. School-based mental health, social and emotional learning, minority mental health, children's mental health, student health

A steady increase in social and related problems has had a negative impact on students' ability to complete school successfully. Changes in family structure, poverty, and economic instability are just a few of the challenges which both weaken families' capacities to care for children and limit their ability to access assistance. Therefore, many children bring problems to school that interfere with learning (Romualdi & Sandoval, 1995). By the fourth grade, the academic performance of most American children is below minimum achievement standards: 75% of students are not proficient in reading, 66% are not proficient in writing, and 82% do not meet appropriate math levels (Carnegie Task Force, 1996). School failure in turn contributes to the rising social problems. According to Comer and Haynes (1995), early school failure is a major predictor of later school, work, and life failure or difficulty, as well as of more severe mental health problems.

There are strong correlations among mental health status, psychological conflict, social problems and educational achievement (Dryfoos, 1993; Comer & Haynes, 1995). Social crises, like homelessness, exposure to violence and drugs, and inadequate adult supervision, contribute to the onset of diagnosable mental health conditions and behavior difficulties (Wagner, 1994). The serious impact of these pressures on children's development is evident in the increasing numbers of school-aged children in need of psychological/psychiatric intervention for stress-induced symptoms such as: depression, hyperactivity and attention deficit disorders, oppositional behaviors, externalizing and conduct disorders, and substance abuse delinquency (Comer & Haynes, 1995). In fact, one out of five youth aged 10 to 18 suffer from a diagnosable mental disorder, and one out of four report symptoms of emotional disorders (Dryfoos, 1993). Children under more psychosocial pressure fare worse in school. Many at-risk students are children with either identified or unidentified behavioral and emotional problems. For example, in Maine, 10% of school dropouts have been identified as having a disorder, and 66% have an unaddressed behavioral or emotional problem (Knitzer et al., 1991).

Children's mental health disorders, including emotional and behavioral problems, have a large social, psychological, cultural, and economic impact on families and communities (Knoff & Batsche, 1990; Osher & Hanley, 1996). Although the problems most visibly and directly affect families with school-aged children, the problem is not limited to them. Society as a whole is paying a price for not intervening in this cycle of social problems that lead to behavioral or emotional difficulties, which in turn lead to school failure, and begin the cycle again. Corporations, for example, are spending $210 billion annually on formal and informal training of poorly educated employees (Peeks, 1993). Hence, the public is essentially financing education twice: once with tax dollars–public and private spending on education is $189 billion (Peeks, 1993)–and again when corporations increase product costs in order to pay for necessary training. Primary prevention and early intervention are clearly much more cost-effective than paying for the consequences of not intervening.

Changes in social, economic, family, and demographic factors demand public schools to do more, yet school standards and services have not changed much in the last 25 years (Carnegie, 1996), so students are unprepared to meet today's challenges. There have been some efforts to address children's social issues and the array of mental health problems which they cause or maintain (Wagner, 1994). Unfortunately, the increase in services has not kept pace with the increase in social stress factors; therefore, the need for services continues to exceed the available resources (Comer & Haynes, 1995).

Although the primary mission of an educational system is academic development, if they are to accomplish educational goals, schools need to assume more responsibility for addressing these social and behavioral issues. Comer and Haynes 1995 (p. 3) noted: "Where underdevelopment or bad development has taken place [in a child] prior to school, schools must support adequate development of experience failure in the promotion of development along cognitive/academic pathways. Most literature supports this contention that social competence and psychological well-being are significantly related to academic achievement; students can learn to the full extent of their abilities if they are under less psychological duress" (Boger, 1990; and Peeks, 1993).

Schools should address students' total development by integrating the input and expertise of significant adults in children's lives. Schools are optimal service delivery sites because of the number of students and families they have the potential to reach. Children are mandated to attend school, and school is really the only common setting remaining for children (Talley & Short, 1996; Dryfoos, 1993; Comer & Haynes, 1996b). This factor helps conquer barriers to service delivery such as time and transportation (Osher & Hanley, 1996), as well as giving care workers access to high-risk, needy populations who would not ordinarily receive services (Dryfoos, 1993). The benefits of this approach extend beyond the immediate care received; they also teach students and families why and how to access services in the future (Dryfoos, 1993).

Schools are also very influential on children's growth because of the amount of time children spend in school. At least half of a child's developmental period is spent in school (Osher & Hanley, 1996; Knoff & Batsche, 1990). Educators need to assume responsibility for the developmental environment that they have direct control over, namely the school setting. School is the first opportunity professionals have to reinforce positive growth and development begun in the community and family or to compensate for underdevelopment (Comer & Haynes, 1995; Knoff & Batsche, 1990; Leaf et al., 1992). This is important because primary caretakers are either failing to recognize treatable problems (Zahner & Pawelkiewiez, 1992) or are unable to handle them.

A school's period of influence is also well timed with children's most important developmental period. This makes the school's role even more important. The long-term success of learning and development largely depends on what happens to a child between the ages of three and 10 (Carnegie, 1996). During this period, it is especially important that children establish a high level of attachment that enables adults to influence their behavior (Comer & Haynes, 1996b). As school demands exceed preparation, and cognitive capacity increases to allow an understanding of social problems, the ability of adults to influence positively children's behavior and aspirations decreases when the child is around the nine years old, if he/she is without attachments (Comer & Haynes, 1996b).

Although schools can have a positive influence on children. They can also have a negative impact if they do not take their responsibility seriously. A child's mental health condition can become aggravated both by interactions in school and by the schooling process (Knoff & Batsche, 1990). School-related stress plays a role in triggering predisposed conditions; the potential for conflict and for psychological stress is high in schools for staff, students, and parents because of the many people involved in the educational process and because of different goals, motivations, and backgrounds of people within the school (Comer & Haynes, 1995). Hence, differences in educational performance are not the result of differences in students' inherent ability to learn. These differences are a culmination of the failure of schools to respond to increasing needs of students who are under more social pressure (Haynes et al., 1993); their low expectations; a heavy reliance on ineffective curricula and teaching methods; poorly prepared, insufficiently supported teams; weak home-school linkages; a lack of accountability systems; and poor resource allocation (Carnegie, 1996).

Educators realize that children are failing, but reform mechanisms have mainly focused on increasing excellence through competency tests and cognitive skills work (Knitzer et al., 1991; Purkey, 1988). This strategy does not help students, especially those at high risk, unless it is accompanied by strong support services (Knitzer et al., 1991). This emphasis on increasing test scores only and neglecting the social and emotional needs of children has caused a neglect of affective education and developmental concerns that affect student growth (Haynes et al., 1993; Purkey, 1988). Reform efforts will be costly and ineffective as long as underlying developmental and social issues remain unaddressed. Despite this fact, neither federal nor local school reform policies have encouraged changes in the educational process that will support the overall development of students and address increasing social challenges (Knoff & Curtis, 1996); Ysseldyke & Geenen, 1996; Haynes et al., 1993).

How should schools address the social problems and psychological stress kids are grappling with? The ecological/systems approach to school reform is the most effective way to support whole child development and to make long-lasting improvements in children's lives. The best way to understand a school and the people within in it is to look at its organizational culture–the guiding beliefs and expectations for how a school operates and how people relate to each other (Thacker, 1994). Most problems and solutions stem from the ecological or systems level, not the individual level; therefore, it is at the systems level where intervention is most effective. Ehly (1993) summarizes the critical assumptions behind the ecological change model:

1. Children are considered to be inseparable parts of the targeted social system,
2. Disturbance is assumed to reflect the system rather than a disease or problem located within the child; the environment can be structured to influence behaviors, and
3. Problems are cast as a failure of match between the child and the system;

Both the abilities of the child and the expectations of the system need to be in line with one another. The end result of the ecological approach as applied to school reform is a successful child-centered, whole school change.

Mental health and support service providers, such as psychologists and social workers, make optimal school change agents within the ecological approach because their professional training gives them the background and skills to implement the child-centered reform processes previously discussed. In order for any system changes to be effective, individuals who have expertise in planning, problem solving, and facilitating organizational change need to be involved in the planning and implementation of changes (Curtis & Stollar, 1996). Psychologists and other support service providers are in the best position to fulfill this need for experts. They should have the skills to be able to sustain broad reform goals while still remaining within their field of expertise, as they target cognitive, affective, and structural components of the school system (Curtis & Stollar, 1996). If the reform goals are student-centered as they should be, schools need to rely on the competencies of counselors regardless of who is implementing the changes (Holcomb & Niffenegger, 1992). Holcomb and Niffenegger (1992) and Ysseldyke and Geenen (1996) cite particular competencies that could be used by counselors. Included are collaborative skills; communication, conflict management, and problem-solving skills; individual and group counseling skills; consulting skills; diagnostic testing skills; and knowledge about child development and social issues.

In order to deliver services in schools effectively, counselors and psychologists need to be comfortable navigating throughout the various systems in which children interact, e.g., family, peer, school, and community systems (Conoley and Conoley, 1991). To act as a school reform facilitator would not require a significant role change for support service providers; it would simply involve applying their work and theoretical orientation to the whole school. Given the connection that exists between behavior, emotion, and learning (Talley & Short, 1996), schools should benefit from applying knowledge of psychology at the community, school, classroom, and individual levels (Riley, 1996). For example, Comer and Haynes (1996b) identified several issues that emerge in school which require knowledge of behavioral and social sciences that psychologists and other support service providers have: school size and architecture, compensatory education programs, issues related to busing and school desegregation, management of trauma, racial identification issues, class and race relations, and gender issues. Other roles have been identified for support service providers to complement their function as behavior and development experts. Behavioral scientists, for example, can promote health-enhancing behavior to prevent many health disorders (Thomas, 1987) and address health disorders that have psychological or environmental roots, e.g., eating disorders (Talley & Short, 1996).

Using their already developed professional skills, support service providers could help students balance academic, social, emotional, and behavioral demands (Holcomb & Niffenegger, 1992; Riley, 1996) while reducing psychosocial dynamics that interfere with learning (Comer & Haynes, 1995). On another level, psychologists and social workers can also provide support to teachers. Service professionals can be used as consultants to help teachers solve problems before they escalate (Riley, 1996); they are crucial agents in structuring, delivering, and evaluating interventions at the classroom level (Ehly, 1993). In particular they can teach school staff

a. how student fears and anxieties influence behavior,
b. how excessive control and punishment worsen behavior,
c. how motivation grows out of the affective component of learning,
d. how staff behaviors dictate student responses,
e. how child development and social conditions factor into learning (Comer & Haynes, 1996b; Comer & Haynes, 1995).

Increasing staff and parent understanding of development and behavior through consultation will improve student behavior and academic performance.

Mental health workers and other support service professionals are currently not being used to their full capabilities. Most continue to follow the tradition of providing adjunct services, marginal to the daily functioning of the school (Lee, 1993). The current, unenlightened system only provides students and families with the necessary attention and access to resources after a problem has escalated out of control (Elias, 1995; Romualdi & Sandoval, 1995). If counselors are going to be of help to educators and students, they need to increase access to both crisis intervention and case management services that are connected to the school life of the child (Knitzer et al., 1992).

Increasingly, the bulk of support service professionals' time has been spent on special education-related tasks. School systems are mandated to provide appropriate educational programs, assessment, and evaluation for special needs children (Thomas, 1987). The unintended result of this federal mandate was a reduction in regular services and attention for the general school population, and a heavy focus on testing and assessment of children with learning, behavioral, or emotional problems.

The role of psychologists in implementation of this act was designed to include assessment and evaluation, consultation, psychological counseling, and parent training, but theory has not manifested itself in practice (Dwyer & Gorin, 1996). Even with its specialized target population the emphasis is not on helping them overcome the behavioral or emotional problems which hinder learning and development. Rather, the emphasis is on altering the educational programming to suit individual learning capabilities. School support personnel quickly refer students with behavioral problems to special education, rather than trying to address the root of the problem through counseling or other interventions (Knitzer et al., 1991).

The extent to which school support professionals have to spend their time doing evaluations and paperwork is being questioned. There is a significant discrepancy between the role stated by school counselors as ideal and the actual role being fulfilled. Ideally, counselors would like to emphasize classroom guidance, parent and faculty workshops, and consulting (Carroll, 1993), but most do not have the time to assume any additional responsibilities. Some school psychologists are participating in Goals 2000, the federal education goals, by assisting with violence prevention programs (Goal 7), improving curriculum and instruction (Goals 3 & 5), and promoting home-school collaboration (Goal 8) (Ysseldyke & Geenen, 1996). These are positive steps, but support personnel are still not being assigned an active role in the school reform process because they are too busy serving a select portion of the school population.

The service delivery system has remained crisis oriented and reactive partially because providers are overwhelmed with demands for services. Fifteen to 19% of US children need mental health care (Wagner, 1994), but at current staffing levels support cannot be provided for all students. Even of those students in most serious need of counseling, only 25-40% are receiving assistance amounting to approximately 22.8 hours per year for each child (Osher & Hanley, 1996). A 1988 national education longitudinal study found that only 11% of eighth graders had had the opportunity to speak to a school counselor or teacher about a personal problem within the last year (Dryfoos, 1993). Empirical research has recommended a caseload of 300 students per school counselor (Carroll, 1993), yet Dryfoos (1993) found that there are approximately 70,000 guidance counselors in public schools which averages to about one counselor per 600 children. One person could certainly not provide adequate individual support for 600 people.

The federal government is not supporting increased support services, either (Dryfoos, 1993; Knitzer et al., 1991), which exacerbates the marginalization of these important mental health and social services within a school. At the state level, only 11 states have legislation mandating elementary school counseling (Bailey et al., 1989). The result is that there are too few support service professionals working in schools to meet demands for health, psychological, and social services (Ehly, 1993), let alone enough to have a lasting impact on the school as a whole (Osher & Hanley, 1996). Fifty-eight percent of schools have no capacity to provide any counseling services (Knitzer et al., 1991).

Support personnel are among the first to be eliminated in budget cuts (Dryfoos, 1993; Adelman, 1996); clearly administrators and communities do not recognize their importance. This is in part because few educators include addressing social problems among the school's responsibilities (Ehly, 1993), or consider themselves in complex social systems (Comer & Haynes, 1995). This has led to a clear separation between education and mental health within the minds of educators. According to Comer and Haynes (1995), this separation is evident at the national, state. and local levels: first, in the lack of cooperation between the National Institute of Mental Health and the National Institute of Education; second, in the lack of cooperation between state departments of education and mental health in service delivery and research; third, in the minimal consultation services and cooperation between mental health workers and educators.

Support service providers are also partially to blame for their insignificant role in the educational system. There is a lack of understanding of the mental health professional's role within the school, so social workers, counselors and school psychologists should do more to define and explain their position (Bailey et al., 1989). Role expectations do vary from district to district depending on needs of the school (Thomas et al., 1992), but there is still too much role confusion (O'Dell et al., 1996) which decreases support for the counselor's services. The general school population is not sure why the social worker works in a certain way, how the approach meets the needs and goals of the school, how decisions are made, and what arrangements exist to maintain accountability (Comer & Haynes, 1995).

Other problems with the delivery system include fragmented and uncoordinated services. Because school service professionals often operate in isolation from each other, they frequently engage in a duplication of efforts or conflicting interventions (Adelman, 1993; Romualdi & Sandoval, 1995). Programs have failed to coordinate services within the school and community and the students have paid the price with inefficient and costly services, as well as a lack of continuity in programming for various problems and across grade levels (Elias, 1995; Adelman, 1993). In one New York school where there were 200 different prevention and treatment programs operating concurrently, even the principal could not identify the function of any of the programs (Dryfoos, 1993). It is less effective to divide problems into strict categories because children often have multiple, interconnected needs (Osher & Hanley, 1996). This concept is not understood by the decision makers, most of whom do not have a counseling background–yet another reason for increasing the role support service providers play in schools.

It is interesting to note that school service use statistics contradict the lack of importance placed on school-based support services. A study by Zahner & Pawelkiewiez (1992) found that in a population of children aged 6-11 years old, 28.3% of the total sample had service contact and 51.2% of the at-risk students had access to services. The overall service use of the sample was considerably larger than estimates for the general child population of 5% and 10-20% respectively (Zahner & Pawelkiewiez, 1992). School service usage accounted for the difference. When service usage was restricted to other settings, the rates of service were comparable to national levels (Zahner & Pawelkiewiez, 1992).

Despite the shortcomings of the current school service system, when programs are well-implemented, funded, and staffed they can be quite effective because of the large numbers of students and families who opt for school services when they are available. Given the extensive use of school mental health and social support services, more importance should be placed on providing adequate services for children within the school setting, and on the role of the support service professionals who work within a school.

Researchers have identified several areas where school support service professionals could expand their influence while using a systems approach and focusing on the whole child. Social reform in education that emphasizes educational achievement, whole-child development, and school climate offers great potential for enhancing the role of the school support staff such as psychologists and social workers. The common denominator of all such reform proposals is collaboration. Multidisciplinary teams composed of counselors, administrators, psychologists, teachers, social workers, and parents are widely supported, especially when the model has the mental health professional acting as the case manager. While the psychologist, for example, would coordinate the group effort, it is important that the input and concerns of each team member carry equal weight. Each team member brings a different perspective to education and this cooperative forum allows members to maximize their individual contributions by making interventions consistent and comprehensive (Thomas, 1987). Such a team meets the requirements for an effective school reform agent; it would enhance classroom-based efforts to enable learning, provide assistance to students and families, prevent crises, support transitions, increase home involvement in schooling, and develop greater community involvement and support (Adelman, 1996).

In districts where a large number of students are underdeveloped, the inevitable high levels of conflict and tension can be reduced by having collaborative management teams that involve administrators, teachers, parents, mental health professionals, and students (Comer & Haynes, 1995). A sample of the characteristics of this team approach which make it effective for improving student outcomes includes: collaborative planning, ownership by the school, the role of the principal, the use of a case manager, shared resources, and staff development (Dolan, 1992). Evidence exists that the case management team approach, under the direction of support service professionals, reduces fragmentation and redundancy of services, increases treatment acceptability, increases generalization of treatment gains, and increases the school's success in managing behavior and learning environments (Conoley & Conoley, 1991). Service delivery also becomes more outcome oriented, consumer driven, and cost conscious (Romualdi & Sandoval, 1995; Shaw et al., 1995), as well as less intimidating and easier to access (Dowling & Taylor, 1989).

The team approach should reduce individuals' respective case loads allowing the professional to dedicate more time and expertise to the school population as a whole. The benefits of this extra time are seen in a team approach advocated by O'Dell et al. (1996), which combines (a) developmental programming aimed at improving the personal, social, and goal planning competencies of all students, (b) preventive programming which targets at-risk students, and (c) remedial programming which serves troubled students. The effects of the program on the school included positive changes in self-concept, a lower failure rate, realistic career planning, higher school functioning, and increased understanding. Clearly, the case management team approach has the greatest impact when there is a commitment to whole-child/whole-school problem solving and an equal focus on individual assessment and systemic issues (Romualdi & Sandoval, 1995; Talley & Short, 1996).

True collaboration also facilitates the development of shared ownership for goal setting and achievement, effective communication, mutual respect, and open-mindedness (Vesey, 1996). Confidence and familiarity with the mental health professional then opens the door for successful consultation at program and organizational levels (Abec, 1987). This level of consultation and collaboration is necessary for systemic change; all major stakeholders must be committed (Curtis & Stollar, 1996). Although systemic change is the end goal, it is important that the team processes be integrated into already existing mechanisms within the school or community; this approach will facilitate a smooth transition, and prohibit cutting back on existing resources (Dryfoos, 1993; Adelman, 1996).

Coordinated services naturally follow from collaboration, since teams will find that no single resource can provide all the services children will need to develop well (Haynes & Comer, 1996). Some schools are now offering children and families a range of services that are centralized under an umbrella organization based either in the school or the community. It is frequently recommended that, in order to satisfy students' diverse needs sufficiently, a comprehensive services network, i.e., including mental health, medical, and social services, needs to be standard for all schools (Dryfoos, 1993). Interdisciplinary service coordination broadens the focus of services, stresses collaboration between many social settings which affect kids, and changes the school's climate (Clancy, 1995). Services should not be limited to mandated services such as special education, but should address the specific needs of a community as determined by the support services team (Romualdi & Sandoval, 1995). All people involved would be part of the decision-making structure.

Several schools have recognized the benefits of physician-psychologist/counselor collaboration because of the reciprocal link among education, social issues, and health. These schools are now successfully applying this model in order to expand their school-based clinics (Talley & Short, 1996; Shaw et al, 1995; Dryfoos, 1993). Talley and Short (1996) found that a truly comprehensive services program must include sequential services in eight different areas: health education, physical education, health services, nutrition services, health promotion, counseling/psychological/social services, a healthy school environment, and parent/community involvement. The expanded role for support service workers would include participation in implementation and administration of services; direct and indirect service provision; interfacing of health and educational outcomes; and research and evaluation (Tharinger, 1995).

According to Haynes and Comer (1996), the entire community benefits from an integrated services approach. Students receive expanded learning opportunities, the attention of caring adults, and increased motivation to stay in school. Families get increased access to social services and an increased ability to network with child development experts and other parents. The school gets a network of services from which to draw support for learning processes.

REFERENCES

Abec, J.M. (1987). Mental health consultation in schools: A developmental perspective. *School Psychology International*, 8(2-3), 73-77.

Adelman, H. (1993). School linked mental health interventions: Toward mechanisms for service coordination and integration. *Journal of Community Psychology*, 21(4), 309-319.

Adelman, H. (1996). Restructuring education support services and integrating community resources: Beyond the full service school model. *School Psychology Review*, 25(4), 431-445.

Bailey, W.R., Deery, N.K., Gehrke, M., & Perry, N. (1989). Issues in elementary school counseling: Discussion with American School Counselor Association Leaders. *Elementary School Guidance & Counseling*, 24(1), 4-13.

Boger, J.M (1990). The mental health team: A process of maximizing human potential in schools. *Paper presented at the annual meeting if the American Educational Research Association.*

Carnegie Task Force on Learning in the Primary Grades (1996). *Years of Promise: A comprehensive learning strategy for America's children.* New York: Carnegie Corporation.

Carroll, B. (1993). Perceived roles and preparation experiences of elementary counselors: Suggestions for change. *Elementary School Guidance & Counseling*, 27, 216-226.

Clancy, J. (1995). Ecological school social work: The reality and the vision. *Social Work in Education*, 17(1), 40-47.

Comer, J.P., & Haynes, N.M., Joyner, E.T., Ben-Avie, M. (Eds.). (1996) *Rallying the whole village: The Comer process for reforming education.* New York: Teachers College Press.

Comer, J.P., & Haynes, N.M. (1996b). Improving psychoeducational outcomes for African American children. *Child and adolescent psychiatry: A comprehensive textbook*, Melvin Lewis (Ed.). Baltimore: Williams & Wilkins, 1097-1103.

Comer, J.P., & Haynes, N.M. (1995). School consultation: A psychosocial perspective. *Psychiatry*, 2(70), 1-13.

Conoley, J., & Conoley, C.W. (1991). Collaboration for child adjustments: Issues for the school and clinic based child psychologists. *Journal of Consulting & Clinical Psychology*, 59(6), 821-829.

Curtis, M.J., & Stollar, S.A. (1996). Applying principles and practices of organizational change to school reform. *School Psychology Review*, 25(4), 409-417.

Dolan, L. (1992). Models for integrating human services into the school. *Johns Hopkins University, Center for Research on Effective Schooling for Disadvantaged Students*, 30.

Dowling, E., & Taylor, D. (1989). The clinic goes to school: Lessons learned. *Maladjustment &Therapeutic Education*, 7(1), 24-29.

Dryfoos, J.G. (1993). Schools as places for health, mental health, and social services. *Teachers College Record*, 94(3), 540-567.

Dryfoos, J.G. (1994). Medical clinics in junior high school: Changing the model to meet demands. *Journal of Adolescent Health*, 15(7), 549-557.

Dwyer, K.P., & Gorin, S. (1996). A national perspective of school psychology in the context of school reform. *School Psychology Review*, 25(4), 507-511.

Ehly, S. (1993). Overview of group intervention for special services providers. *Special Services in School*, 8(1), 9-38.

Elias, M.J. (1995). Primary, prevention as health and social competence promotion. *Journal of Primary Prevention,* 16(8), 5-24.

Emmons, C., Owen, S., Haynes, N., & Comer, J.P. (1992). A causal model of the effects of school climate, classroom climate, academic self-concept, suspension, and absenteeism on academic achievement. *Paper presented at the 1992 conference of the Eastern Educational Research Association.*

Felber, R.D., Aber, M.S., Primavera, J., & Cause, A.M. (1985). Adaptation and vulnerability in high-risk adolescents: An examination of environmental mediators. *American Journal of Community Psychology*, 13(4), 365-379.

Gersch, I., & Noble, J. (1991). A systems project involving students and staff in a secondary school. *Educational Psychology in Practice*, 7(3), 140-147.

Griffith, J. (1995). An empirical examination of a model of social climate in elementary schools. *Basic and Applied Social Psychology*, 17 (I & 2), 97-117.

Haynes, N.M., & Comer, J.P. (1996). Integrating schools, families, and communities through successful school reform: The school development program. *School Psychology Review*, 25(4), 501-506.

Haynes, N.M., Comer, J.P., & Roberts, V. (1993). A developmental and systems approach to mental health in schools. *Educational Horizons*, 71(4), 181-186.

Hertz-Lazarowitz, R., & Cohen, M. (1992). The school psychologist as a facilitator of a community-wide project to enhance positive learning climate in elementary schools. *Psychology in Schools*, 29(4), 348-358.

Holcomb, T., & Niffenegger, P.B. (1992). Elementary school counselors: A plan for marketing their services under the new education reforms. *Elementary School Guidance & Counseling*, 27, 56-63.

Indramma, V., & Balasubramanyam, K.K. (1989). A follow-up study on the efficacy of social work intervention in schools. *Child Psychiatry Quarterly*, 22(2-3), 47-50.

Jones, R.A. (1995). *The child-school interface: Environment and behavior*. New York, NY: Cassell.

Kasen, S., Johnson, J., & Cohen, P. (1990). The impact of school emotional climate on student psychopathology. *Journal of Abnormal Child Psychology*, 18(2), 165-178.

Kerwin, C. (1995). Consultation models revisited: A practitioner's perspective. *Journal of Educational & Psychological Consultation*, 6(4), 373-383.

Knitzer, J., Steinburg, Z., & Fleisch, B. (1991). Schools, children's mental health, and the advocacy challenge. Special Issue: Child Advocacy. *Journal of Clinical Child Psychology*, 20(1), 102-111.

O'Dell, F.L., Rak, C.F., Chermonte, J.P., Hamlin, A., & Waina, N. (1996). Guidance for the 1990's: Revitalizing the counselor's role. *The Clearing House*, 69(5), 303-307.

Osher, D., & Hanley, T. (1996). Implications of the national agenda to improve results for children and youth with or at risk of serious emotional disturbance. *Special Services in School*, 7-35.

Osterweil, Z.O. (1988). A structured integrative model of mental health consultation in schools. *International Journal for the Advancement of Counseling*, II *(1), 37-49.*

Peeks, B. (1993). Revolutions in counseling and education: A systems perspective in the schools. *Elementary School Guidance & Counseling*, 27, 245-251.

Purkey, W.,& Aspy, D.N. (1988). The mental health of students: Nobody minds? Nobody cares? *Person-Centered Review*, 3(1), 41-49.

Reynolds, D. (1987). The effective school: Do educational psychologists help or hinder? *Educational Psychology in Practice*, 3(3), 22-28.

Riley, R. (1996). Improving America's schools. *School Psychology Review*, 25(4), 477-484.

Roeser, R.W., Midgley, C., & Urdan, T.C. (1996). Perceptions of the school psychological environment and early adolescents' psychological and behavioral functioning in school: The mediating role of goals and belonging. *Journal of Educational Psychology*, 88(3), 408-422.

Romualdi, V. & Sandoval, J. (1995). Comprehensive school-linked services: Implications for school psychologists. *Psychology in the Schools*, 32, 306-317.

Schultz, E.W., Glass, R.M., & Kamholtz, D. (1987). School climate: Psychological health and well-being in school. *Journal of School Health*, 57(10), 432-437.

Shaw, S.R., Kelly, D.P., Joost, J.C., & Parker-Fisher, S.J. (1995). School-linked and schoolbased health services: A renewed call for collaboration between school psychologists and medical professionals. *Psychology in Schools*, 32(3), 190-201.

Sigston, A., Noble, J., Fuller, A., & O'Donaghue, S. (1989). Doing time or negotiating the effective use of educational psychologists' time. *Educational & Child Psychology*, 6(4, pt 2), 39-44.

Stratford, R. (1990). Creating a positive school ethos. *Educational Psychology in Practice*, 5(4), 183-191.

Talley, R.C., & Short, R.J. (1996). Schools as health delivery sites: Current status and future directions. *Special Services in School*, 37-55.

Talley, R.C., & Short, R.J. (1996). Social reforms and the future of school practice: Implications of American psychology. *Professional Psychology: Research and Practice*, 27(1), 5-14.

Thacker, J. (1994). Organizational cultures: How to identify and understand them. *Educational & Child Psychology*, II *(3),* 11-21.

Tharinger, D. (1995). Roles for psychologists in emerging models of school related health and mental health services. *School Psychology Quarterly*, 10(3), 203-216.

Thomas, A. (1987). School psychologist: An integral member of the school health team. *Journal of School Health,* 57(10), 465-469.

Thomas, A., Orf, M., Levinson, E., & Pinciotti, D. (1992). Administrators' perceptions of school psychologists' roles and satisfaction with school psychologists. *Psychological Reports,* 71, 571-575.

Vesey, J. (1996). Team collaboration leads to a sense of community. *NASSP Bulletin,* 80(584), 31-35.

Wagner, W.G. (1994). Counseling with children: An opportunity for tomorrow. *Counseling Psychologist,* 22(3), 381-401.

Weinberg, R.B. (1989). Consultation and training with school-based crisis teams. *Professional Psychology: Research and Practice,* 20(5), 305-308.

Werthamer-Larsson, L. (1994). Methodological issues in school based services research. Special Section: Mental health services research with children, adolescents, and their families. *Journal of Clinical Child Psychology,* 23(2), 121-132.

Ysseldyke, J., & Geenen, K. (1996). Integrating the special education and compensatory education systems into the school reform process: A national perspective. *School Psychology Review,* 25(4), 418-430.

Zahner, G.E., Pawelkiewicz, W., DeFrancesco, J., & Adnopoz, J. (1992). Children's Mental health service needs and utilization patterns in an urban community: An epidemiological assessment. *Journal of the American Academy of Child & Adolescent Psychiatry,* 31(5), 951-960.

Zaki, M., & Partok-Engel, R. (1984). School as agent for mental health socialization of the individual. *School Psychology International,* 5(3), 147-150.

Zins, J.E., Conyne, R.K., & Charlene, R. (1988). Primary prevention: Expanding the impact of psychological services in schools. *School Psychology Review,* 17(4), 542-549.

Parent-Adolescent Interaction: Influence on the Academic Achievement of African American Adolescent Males

Sherin A. Shearin, DSW

SUMMARY. As the achievement gap between African American and white students persists, an examination of factors outside the school setting are essential. Acknowledging the dynamics of family environment as perceived by African American adolescent males is apposite to understanding the relationship between family environment and academic achievement. Utilizing an ecological perspective, this study describes the characteristics of family process variables and analyzes the adolescents' perception of parent-adolescent interaction and its influence on their psychological well-being. Results indicate that a substantial proportion of the 179 adolescent males who perceived parent-adolescent interaction as positive and were identified as having a stable psychological well-being, were more likely to have average to above-average grade point averages, high Stanford Nine scores and high achievement group membership, than those adolescent males who did not perceive parent-adolescent interaction as positive. *[Article copies available for a fee from The Haworth Document Delivery Service: 1-800-HAWORTH. E-mail address: <docdelivery@haworthpress.com> Website: <http://www.HaworthPress.com> © 2002 by The Haworth Press, Inc. All rights reserved.]*

Sherin A. Shearin is affiliated with Norfolk Public School System in Norfolk Virginia as Lead School Social Worker and Adjunct Faculty at the Ethelyn R. Strong School of Social Worker, Norfolk State University, Norfolk, VA.

[Haworth co-indexing entry note]: "Parent-Adolescent Interaction: Influence on the Academic Achievement of African American Adolescent Males." Shearin, Sherin A. Co-published simultaneously in *Journal of Health & Social Policy* (The Haworth Press, Inc.) Vol. 16, No. 1/2, 2002, pp. 125-137; and: *Disability and the Black Community* (ed: Sheila D. Miller) The Haworth Press, Inc., 2002, pp. 125-137. Single or multiple copies of this article are available for a fee from The Haworth Document Delivery Service [1-800-HAWORTH, 9:00 a.m. - 5:00 p.m. (EST). E-mail address: getinfo@haworthpress.com].

http://www.haworthpress.com/store/product.asp?sku=J045
10.1300/J045v16n01_11

KEYWORDS. Parent-adolescent interaction, academic achievement, family environment, family process, psychological well-being

One of the greatest challenges for African American students, especially African American males, is the achievement gap that exists between them and their white counterparts. Just how well they fare when compared to students of the dominant race is a question whose answers have been based in negative assumptions and stereotypes. Despite efforts of federally-funded tutorial programs in reading and math, after-school tutoring, and tutoring services provided by local churches, the achievement gap persists. However, much of the empirical research is rendering substantive evidence which indicates that family environments, demographic effects, student attitude, and educational expectations have the largest effects on academic performance and standardized test scores. Notwithstanding that children's academic performance is determined by multiple factors, researchers have been particularly interested in how school functioning is related to family environments (Kurdek & Sinclair, 1988).

Many authors have focused on numerous negative factors and conditions facing our African American adolescent males since the Nation at Risk report of 1983 (National Commission on Excellence in Education, 1983). This report described the adolescents of the 1990s as being in a period of great risk for healthy development. According to Takanishi (1993), school failure or underachievement may co-occur with problems such as drugs, mental disorders, sexual activity, family-related issues, and juvenile delinquency. These educational at-risk symptoms are even more pervasive among African American and minority male youth (Thornburg, Hoffman, & Remeika, 1991). Social science researchers have found that all children do not come to school with the same experiences and preparations to learn; as a result, many minority students, especially African American males, are still not able to measure up academically to their white counterparts.

According to Mann (1997), educators have also been convinced that there are factors outside the school setting influencing the student's achievement. She suggests these factors may include, but are not limited to, biological, sociocultural, psychological, economic, and environmental explanations for the consistent and disturbing findings that the academic performance of many African American male students falls behind that of other groups (1997).

Based on pertinent theories and research findings in the literature, life experiences and psychological well-being are affected by the conditions of the child's environment and learning is dependent in part on these two elements. Psychological well-being also comprised of these characteristics lends itself to what the child perceives as a stable peace of mind and a supportive family environment. When children are raised in a home that nurtures a sense of self-worth, competence, well-being and autonomy, children will be more apt to accept the risks inherent in learning. These elements are essential to the socialization process and psychological well-being of African American children if they are to survive and become productive citizens.

The question confronting most social workers, educators, psychologists, and researchers is how do we account for the differences in children's academic performance? Is there something wrong with poor children and children of color, their genes or their families, that undermine their development and achievement (Bowman, 1994)?

Noteworthy is Bowman's (1994) explanation that the difference in school performance lies in the differences in life experiences between groups. The world in which children of diverse cultural and socioeconomic groups live does not always emphasize the same skills. However, the range of adaptive and learning capabilities of minority and poor children is as broad as other children's, posits Bowman (1994). Bowman also notes that schools have ignored or rejected different cultural expressions of development that are normal and adequate and on which school skills and knowledge can be built. She further notes that when public schools ignore the differences between children, they limit their own ability to adequately educate these children (1994). African American children learn to establish and verify perceptions and beliefs about the world through direct teaching by their parents, older people in their families and communities, and through identification with those people who care for them and are emotionally important to them (Delpit, 1988).

Cultural patterns and family interactions guide the developing child, but they also become the basis for the child's definition of self, his or her psychological well-being (Ellison, 1990), and his or her place in society. Though some children are at risk for abnormal development because of deprivations inherent in living in poverty or in crisis-ridden families, most minority and poor children are developmentally normal and their families ably carry out the essential child-rearing functions (Hines & Boyd-Franklin, 1996). Among the primary conditions creating risk factors associated with lower educational achievement are poverty, lack of family guidance, and an unstable psychological well-being.

Family environment as a non-school related factor of academic achievement is the primary social system for children (Dekovics & Janssens, 1992) producing a multilateral influence on their academic performance. Dave (1963) found that family environment influences the extent of children's educational growth directly by determining the nature and quality of the educative experiences, exerting a relatively less direct influence on children's educational process, therefore, stimulating their capacity to learn. As the primary source of socialization, family interaction, life experiences to include family and community influences, shapes the initial constellation of attitudes children develop toward education (DeKovics & Janssens, 1992). These attitudes are dependent upon the experience and intent of the mediating adult who frames, selects, focuses, and interprets the experiences for children in ways that produce the culturally appropriate educative style (Feuerstein, 1979).

The socialization experience of most African American children found in traditional African American families has a foundation of nurturing and support, joined by an Afrocentric instruction of a committed love of family, mutual cooperation and responsibility, and the formation of a racial identity (Prince, 1997). Of even more significance for African American adolescent males is that negative educational outcomes have substantial social and economic costs for those at-risk as well as a significant impact on society (Thornburg, et al., 1991). Labor force projections are indicating a serious decline in the number of blue collar jobs and a substantial increase in jobs requiring high-level technical skills (Denbow, 1997). Given this economic picture, the crisis of underachieving African American male students is becoming a critical issue in determining our nation's economic survival.

Research is suggesting family interactions to be particularly important to the psychological well-being of children manifested by (1) parental support and encouragement of positive attitudes toward education, (2) high expectation for student success, and (3) parental involvement in the schools as having a profoundly positive effect on academic achievement (Ellison, 1990; Hess & Holloway, 1985). Whereas, when children do not view self as basically competent and able, and their psychological well-being at risk, freedom to engage in academically challenging pursuits and the capacity to tolerate and cope with failure are greatly diminished (Lumsden, 1994). There has been a general inconsistency in results of numerous studies on the above-stated premise operating under the perception that African American families are monolithic (Scott-Jones, 1984).

According to Scott-Jones (1984), these inconsistencies originated from invalid assumptions made about the nature and role of home environmental factors, invalid assumptions about group homogeneity stemming from a lack of understanding of the differences that exist among and within minority groups, and the assumption that environmental factors are static factors and can be isolated for analysis. To the contrary, these factors are not static, they operate in an interactive fashion with each other and with other social factors within the larger societal context.

African American families have a history of being strong, functional, and flexible (Hill, 1971; Billingsley, 1968). They provide a home environment that is culturally different from that of Euro-American families in several ways. Of significance, is that the family environment of African Americans is described as including not only the special stress of poverty or of discrimination, but the ambiguity and marginality of living simultaneously in two worlds: the world of the Black community and the world of mainstream society, a phenomenon unique to African Americans for many decades.

Researchers and theorists addressing parent-child interactive relations have repeatedly made reference to two broad dimensions of interaction. In earlier studies, Maccoby and Martin (1983), and Argyle and Henderson (1985) organized parent-child interaction on the basis of two dimensions. The particular labels varied from author to author, yet one dimension consistently refers to levels of emotional support provided by parents to their children. The dimension of parental support appears to be related to socially valued characteristics of children including advanced cognitive ability, academic success, psychological well-being, and high self-esteem. Supportive behavior was characterized as

1. expressing interest in children's activities,
2. talking with children,
3. taking children on outings or playing games with them,
4. providing help with everyday problems or schoolwork,
5. expressing enthusiasm and praise over their accomplishments, and
6. showing affection and love (Argyle & Henderson, 1985; Maccoby & Martin, 1983).

Dave (1963), out of the University of Chicago, did his doctoral dissertations on family environmental factor's relationship to academic achievement of white middle-class students. He hypothesized that parental behaviors and parent-child interactive behavior are most likely to foster intellectual growth. These findings were later supported in the works of Ketsetzis, Ryan, and Adams (1998), and Moos (1994), who agree that interactive behaviors constitute the educational environment in the home from which the child takes his cue.

In order to describe the phenomenon linking family process factors to academic achievement, an ecological perspective approach was selected. An ecological perspective encompasses an examination of several dimensions of the environment (Greene & Barnes, 1998). It is concerned with the interaction, transaction, and interrelationships between the individual and the environment (Greene, 1999). The ecological perspective best supports looking at multiple variables within the many dimensions of family systems, integrating knowledge from many different sources.

Chestang, one of the forerunners of ecological perspective, applied the interrelatedness of societal factors and individual factors as it impacts on African Americans and their environments (Greene & Barnes, 1998). Bronfenbrenner

(1989) expanded on the ecological perspective in his conceptualization that ecological theory is a process of the individual in context. He describes four levels of systems that influence individuals and their functioning in society: microsystem, mesosystem, exosystem, and macrosystem. When applied to this research study, the various system levels include the effects of the socialization process and psychological well-being, interactions between the adolescent and parent, the influence of parental support and encouragement, achievement oriented activities, and the indirect impact of parents' employment and the culture of the dominant society.

External systems likely to impinge on the reality of African American families, particularly family process, impact the child's perception of self, his capability, and his interaction with the family and other social systems. The child's perception of the family's positive interaction and support frames his psychological well-being (Ellison, 1990) which enhances his self-efficacy. These attributes help to guide the child in academic pursuits. According to Bandura (1993), perceived self-efficacy is concerned with judgements of how well one can execute courses of action required to deal with prospective situations.

Zimmerman (1995) noted that initial efficacy experiences are centered in the family. As the child reaches adolescence, the ease with which the transition from childhood to adolescence is made depends on the assurance in one's capabilities built up through prior experiences. Experiences from years of parental support, encouragement, and confidence that a task set before the child can be mastered is undergirded by the praises and support for similar situations from people important in the child's life. This is manifested in the use of verbal persuasion by parents of the child's capability to master a given task. However, persuasive appraisals should be weighed in terms of who the persuader is and how credible the persuader is in terms of how knowledgeable they are about the nature of the activity to be undertaken (Horn, Bruning, Schraw, Curry, & Katkanant, 1993).

The more believable the source of persuasion, the more likely are judgements of personal efficacy and the more likely the individual is to mobilize greater sustained effort toward mastering a task, than if there had been no such experiences (Horn et al., 1993). Consequently, self-efficacy beliefs affect motivation to learn, hence, improved academic attainment.

What the adolescent brings to the educational environment contributes to his perception and judgement of his capabilities to perform academically. Adolescents who are more self-efficacious are more apt to experience successful outcomes. Efficacy of academic achievement does occur in those students who perceive their own psychological well-being as positive based on a family environment that is nurturing, supportive, achievement-oriented and encourages educational attainment (Bandura, 1993).

METHOD

The present quantitative research study is descriptive in nature in that it describes the relationship between family process variables, as perceived by the adolescent and parent, and the academic achievement of African American adolescent males. This study utilized an African American research model which views African Americans as normative for African Americans. According to Akbar (1981), the diverse occurrence of African American people in a wide variety of social, economic, political, and cultural environments produces a broad base for providing meaningful information about variables of similarity among this ethnic group.

Sampling Procedure

A stratified random sample based on ethnic group membership (African American), grade (7th and 8th), and birth year (between 1985 and 1987) was obtained from the school. Letters explaining the research study and informed consent forms were mailed to all eligible African American male students. Of the 230 letters and consent forms mailed to the parents of the students, 179 students who returned signed parent consent forms constituted the study sample population. Participation was voluntary for students and parents.

Instruments

Data pertaining to parent-adolescent interaction was collected using two instruments. The Demographic Family Profile (DFP) developed by Shearin (1997) used to obtain parents' perception of their involvement with their adolescent and his school has 13 items to assess the extent to which parents perceive their support and encouragement toward their adolescents' academic success. Parents were asked to select the answer from a list of possible answers that most closely described their involvement with their adolescents' education. Three subscales of the Family Environment Scale (FES) developed by R. H. Moos and B. S. Moos (1974) were used to assess the extent to which adolescents perceive their family/social environments. It is a 90-item scale written in a true/false format clustered under three dimensions.

Relationship Dimension:

1. Cohesion,
2. Expressiveness, and
3. Conflict.

Personal Growth Dimension:

   4. Independence,
   5. Achievement Orientation,
   6. Intellectual-Cultural Orientation,
   7. Active-Recreational Orientation, and
   8. Moral-Religious Emphasis.

System Maintenance Dimension:

   9. Organization, and
  10. Control.

The three subscales most closely linked to child competence and academic achievement, Cohesion (COH), Achievement Orientation (AO), and Intellectual-Cultural Orientation (ICO) (Moos, 1994), were used in the analysis.

Academic achievement was operationalized using participants' combined grade point average (GPA) from two consecutive semesters of the 1999-2000 school year. Participants' stanine scores from the Stanford Nine Achievement Test (STAN 9) were also used as a construct of academic achievement.

RESULTS

A total of 179 African American middle school adolescent males completed the FES. Of the total participants, 46.9 percent were 7th graders and 53.1 percent were 8th graders; the mean age was thirteen years, five months (13-5). One-hundred-and-two participants were from two-parent households and 68 were from mother-only headed households. A total of 178 parents completed the DFP questionnaire; one parent declined to participate.

Participants were divided into two achievement groups: 63.1 percent of the participants were in the high achievers group with a GPA of 2.50 or better and low achievement group membership was comprised of those participants, 36.9 percent, with a GPA of 2.49 or lower. The GPA is based on a 4.0 equals A grading scale. The mean GPA obtained was 2.65 with a standard deviation of .5055. Stanine scores were obtained for the Stanford Nine Achievement Test, average stanine scores ranging between 4 and 6; the mean Stanford Nine Score obtained was 5.53 with a standard deviation of 1.54.

A Pearson's correlation determined that there was a significant association between family process variables of "parent helps with homework" ($r = .45$), "achievement orientation" ($r = .80$), and "intellectual-cultural orientation" ($r = .82$) at $p < .01$, and participants' academic achievement. "Family cohesion" was significant ($r = -.16$) at the $p < .05$ level of significance. These correlations warranted further analysis using stepwise multiple regression to determine the strength of the relationships. When the variables (a) at least one parent has met child's teacher, etc. (SCHCONT), (b) son does homework (HOMWRK), (c) parent helps with homework (PHLPHMWRK), (d) family resources (RESOURCE), (e) family cohesion (COH), (f) achievement orientation (AO), and (g) intellectual-cultural orientation (ICO) were entered into the regression equation, ICO entered first, followed by AO and then COH and PHLPHMWRK. These results indicate that Intellectual-Cultural Orientation accounted for 82 percent of the variance in participants' GPAs and Achievement Orientation explained 3 percent of the variance. Cohesion contributed an additional 3 percent to the variance of participants' GPAs while only 1 percent of the variance was contributed by " parent helps with homework."

To determine which of the variables assessing parent-adolescent interaction have the greatest predictive power of participants' GPAs, an examination of the magnitude of the beta coefficients revealed ICO ($B = .82$, $p < .0001$) to have the greatest predictive power of the three variables. A summary of the results of stepwise regression predicting participants' GPAs from three subscales of the FES along with variables from the DFP is presented in Table 1.

Variables identified above from the DFP were those variables most likely to be associated with adding to the adolescents' psychological well-being. A stepwise regression analysis was performed with these variables being regressed on participants' GPAs. It was noted that 30 percent of the variance of participants' GPAs could be explained by son does homework regularly (HOMWRK). Parent helps with homework (PHLPHMWRK) contributed an additional 2 percent of the variance. To further determine the extent of the relationship, an examination of the magnitude of the beta coefficients revealed "son does homework regularly" to have the greatest predictive power ($B = .55$, $p < .0001$) of participants' GPAs as presented in Table 2. "Educational resources available in the home" and "parental contact with school personnel," noted as being important to academic achievement in the literature (Chapman, Lambourne, & Silva, 1990; Rosenthal & Feldman, 1991; Wentzel, 1994), showed no statistically significant effect on participants' academic achievement when entered into a regression equation.

Next, a stepwise multiple regression was performed regressing all of the variables identified from the FES and the DFP with participants' Stanford 9 Achievement scores. Achievement Orientation explained 54 percent of the variance in participants' Stanford 9 scores. An additional 3 percent of the variance was accounted for by ICO and 1 percent was explained by both COH and PHLPHMWRK. An examination of the magnitude of the beta coefficients found AO ($B = .73$, $p < .0001$) to have the greatest predictive power of participants' Stanford 9 scores. It has been shown through stepwise multiple regression that there is a positive relationship between parent-adolescent interaction and participants' academic achievement, with strong statistically significant

TABLE 1. Summary of Stepwise Regression Analysis of Parent-Adolescent Interaction Variables Predicting Participants' GPAs (N = 179)

Variables[a]	B	$SE\ B$	B
Step 1			
ICO	.23	.01	.82****
Step 2			
ICO	.14	.02	.49****
AO	.11	.02	.38****
Step 3			
ICO	.14	.02	.51****
AO	.11	.02	.36****
COH	−4.089E-02	.00	−.17****
Step 4			
ICO	.14	.02	.51****
AO	9.483E-02	.02	.30****
COH	−4.183E-02	.00	−.17
PHLPHMWRK	6.461E-02	.02	.13

Note. R-square = .67 for Step 1; R-square Change = .03 for Step 2; $p < .0001$;
a. RESOURCE, SCHCONT, and HOMWRK, were excluded from the equation;
****$p < .0001$

predictive powers, when measured using two distinct indices of participants' academic achievement.

DISCUSSION

The importance of the adolescents' perception of family environment is a vital factor of their psychological well-being even though very subjective when considering the influence it may have on the adolescents' academic achievement. How the participant perceives family interaction, support, commitment, and involvement helps to enhance his psychological well-being and how he believes himself to be capable of performing successfully academically. The subjective image of family relationships provides one perspective through which to view the dynamics of the relationship between family environment, the adolescent, and academic achievement. Academic achievement defined as the result of positive effort expended by the student to perform successfully in those subjects undertaken in school is framed by the student's self-efficacy. Much of the effort in self-efficacy is derived from the student's psychological well-being, his peace of mind that family relationships are good

TABLE 2. Summary of Stepwise Regression of DFP Variables Predicting Participants' GPAs

Variables[a]	B	SE B	B
Step 1			
HOMWRK	.41	.04	.55****
Step 2			
HOMWRK	.33	.05	.43****
PHLPHMWRK	9.240-02	.03	.19****

Note R-square = .30 for Step 1, $p < .0001$; *R*-square Change = .02 for Step 2, $p < .01$.
a. RESOURCE and SCHCONT were excluded from the equation;
***$p < .001$, ****$p < .0001$

and positive and supportive. How well an individual thinks himself capable of performing successfully, completing a task, or achieving high grades is based in part on his psychological well-being.

When the participants were grouped according to high and low achievers, 76.7 percent of the high achievers perceived family support, commitment, encouragement, and help to be rated between average and considerably above average. Being exposed to achievement oriented and intellectual-cultural oriented activities was also rated between average and considerably above average by 94.2 percent of the high achievers. Parents also saw themselves as being supportive and involved with their adolescents' educational performance as demonstrated in the results of stepwise regression analysis.

One of the expectations of this study was that the African American adolescent male can experience academic success when his psychological well-being is stable/good and he perceives himself as being a member of a family environment that is positive, interactive, and supportive. Chapman, Lambourne, and Silva (1990) found, in the context of high family support, an emphasis on achievement and structure typically leads to better academic performance.

CONCLUSION

It can be concluded from the data presented above that African American adolescent middle school males' academic achievement is significantly related to family process variables. Participants' perception of positive parent-adolescent interaction which supports a stable sense of psychological well-being enhances their efforts toward high academic achievement. The findings suggest that family process variables and participants' academic achievement are interrelated. Inherent in these findings is the notion that the participants' academic performance may be enhanced or hindered by a stable or unstable psychological well-being and a positive or negative perception of their interactions with their parents. Psychological well-being and positive perceptions are reflected in how capable the adolescent believes himself to be and how motivated he is to perform successfully in the academic arena. The statistically significant findings of positive parent-adolescent interactions add to the knowledge of family process variables as predictors of participants' academic achievement.

This newly acquired knowledge should lead to the development of specific and effective interventions designed to improve academic achievement through the involvement of family environments. These findings further suggest that effort should be made by social work practitioners and school social workers, in particular, to bridge the gap between school systems, families, and policy-makers in an effort to promote family environments that are warm, structured, interactive, and supportive; family environments that will enhance a stable psychological well-being for children in order for them to actively improve their academic achievement.

REFERENCES

Akbar, N. (1981). Paradigms of African American research. In R. L. Jones (Ed.), *Black Psychology, (3rd ed)*. Berkeley, CA: Cobb & Henry.

Argyle, M. & Henderson, M. (1985). *The anatomy of relationships*. Harmondsworth, Middlesex, England: Penguin.

Bandura, A. (1993). Perceived self-efficacy in cognitive development and functioning. *Educational Psychologist, 28*, 117-148.

Billingsley, A. (1968). *Black families in white America*. New York: Simon & Schuster, Inc.

Bowman, B. J. (1994). Cultural diversity and academic achievement. NCREL's Urban Education Program. A Monograph.

Bronfenbrenner, U. (1989). Ecological systems theory. *Annals of Child Development, 6*, 187-249.

Chapman, J. W., Lambourne, R., & Silva, P. A. (1990). Some antecedents of academic self concept: A longitudinal study. *British Journal of Educational Psychology, 60*,142-152.

Dave, R. (1963). *The identification and measurement of environmental process variables that are related to educational environment*. Unpublished doctoral dissertation, University of Chicago.

DeKovics, M. & Janssens, J.M.A.M. (1992). Parent's child rearing style and child's sociometric status. *Developmental Psychology, 28* (5), 925-932.

Delpit, L. D. (1988). The silenced dialogue: Power and pedagogy in educating other people's children. *Harvard Educational Review, 58*, 280-298.

Denbow, S. (1997). Cross-cultural communication. Northwest Regional Education laboratory, Portland, OR.

Ellison, G. G. (1990). Family ties, friendships, and subjective well-being among Black Americans. *Journal of Marriage and the Family, 32,* 290-310.

Feuerstein, R. (1979). *The dynamic assessment of retarded performers.* Baltimore, MD: University Park Press.

Greene, R. R. & Barnes, G. (1998). The ecological perspective, diversity and culturally competent social work practice. In R. R Greene & M. Watkins (Eds.), *Serving diverse constituencies: Applying the ecological perspective.* New York: Aldine De Gruyer.

Hess, R. & Holloway, S. (1985). Family and school as educational institutions. In R. Parke (Ed.), *Review of child development research.* Chicago: University of Chicago Press.

Hill, R. (1971). *The strengths of Black families.* New York: Emerson-Hall.

Hines, P. M. & Boyd-Franklin, N. (1996). African American families. In M. McGoldrick, J. Giordano, & J. Pearce (Eds), *Ethnicity and family therapy* (2nd ed.), (pp 68-84). New York: The Guilford Press.

Ketsetzis, M., Ryan, B. A., & Adams, G. R. (1998). Family process, parent-child interaction, and child characteristics influencing school-based social adjustment. *Journal of Marriage and the Family, 60,* 374-387.

Kremer, B. K. & Walberg, H. (1981). A synthesis of social and psychological influence on science learning. *Science Education, 65,* 11-23.

Kurdek, L. A. & Sinclair, R. J. (1988). Relation of eighth grader's family structure, gender, and family environment with academic performance and school behavior. *Journal of Educational Psychology, 80* (1), 90-94.

Leicht, H. J. (1984). Families as environment for literacy. In H. O. Goelman, A. Oberg, & F. Smith (Eds.), *Awakening to Literacy.* Exeter, NH: Heinemann Educational Books.

Lumsden, L. S. (1994). *Student motivation to learn,* ERIC Digest, 92.

Maccoby, E. E. & Martin, J., (1983). Socialization in the context of the family: Parent-child interaction. In E. M. Hetherington (Ed.) & P. H. Mussen (Series Ed.) *Handbook of child psychology: Socialization, personality, and social development.* Vol. 4 (pp 1-101), New York: Wiley.

Mann, T. (1997). Profile of African Americans, 1970-1995. *The Black Collegian Magazine.* Black Collegiate Services, Inc. Washington, DC: Urban Institute.

Moos, R. H. & Moos, B. S. (1994). Family Environment Scale Manual (3rd ed.). Palo Alto, CA: Consulting Psychologists Press.

Moos, R. H. (1974). Family Environment Scale (Form R). Palo Alto, CA: Consulting Psychologists Press, Inc.

National Commission on Excellence in Education (1983). *A nation at risk.* Washington, DC: U.S. Government Printing Office.

Prince, K. J. (1997). Black family and Black liberation. *Psychological Discourse, 28* (1), 4-7.

Scott-Jones, D. (1984). Family influences on cognitive development and school achievement. *Review of Research in Education, 11,* 259-306.

Shearin, S. A. (1997). Family Demographic Profile. Norfolk State University, Norfolk, VA.

Takanishi, R. (1993). The opportunities of adolescence research, interventions, and policy. *American Psychologist, 48,* 85-87.

Thornburg, K. R., Hoffman, S., & Remeika, C. (1991). Youth at risk: Society at risk. *The Elementary School Journal, 91,* 199-208.

Zimmerman, B. J. (1995). Self-efficacy and educational development. In A. Bandura, *Self-efficacy in changing societies.* Cambridge: Cambridge University Press.

The State of Mental Health Services for Children and Adolescents: An Examination of Programs, Practices and Policies

Annie Woodley Brown, DSW

SUMMARY. This article presents an overview of the state of mental health services for children and adolescents. It provides a brief historical review of policies affecting mental health services for children and adolescents with emotional and behavioral disorders. It discusses the roles of various systems in the provision services for emotionally and behaviorally disordered children and adolescents, and the need for cross-systems collaboration and funding. A model psycho-educational day treatment program, City Lights, is highlighted as an approach to serving inner-city African American adolescents with a profile of services and of the types of youth best served by such a program. *[Article copies available for a fee from The Haworth Document Delivery Service: 1-800-HAWORTH. E-mail address: <docdelivery@haworthpress.com> Website: <http://www.HaworthPress.com> © 2002 by The Haworth Press, Inc. All rights reserved.]*

KEYWORDS. Mental health services, adolescents, collaboration, emotionally and behaviorally disordered, psycho-education programs

Annie Woodley Brown is Associate Professor, Howard University, School of Social Work.

[Haworth co-indexing entry note]: "The State of Mental Health Services for Children and Adolescents: An Examination of Programs, Practices and Policies." Brown, Annie Woodley. Co-published simultaneously in *Journal of Health & Social Policy* (The Haworth Press, Inc.) Vol. 16, No. 1/2, 2002, pp. 139-153; and: *Disability and the Black Community* (ed: Sheila D. Miller) The Haworth Press, Inc., 2002, pp. 139-153. Single or multiple copies of this article are available for a fee from The Haworth Document Delivery Service [1-800-HAWORTH, 9:00 a.m. - 5:00 p.m. (EST). E-mail address: docdelivery@ haworthpress.com].

Studies indicate that 14%-20% of American children have one or more psychiatric disorders in the moderate to severe range (Kelleher & Wolraich, 1996) and may have a diagnosable mental health disorder (CMHS, 2001). An estimated 4.5 to 6.3 million children in the United States have a serious emotional disturbance (Friedman, Katz-Leavy, Manderschied, & Sondheimer, 1996) and one in 10 suffer from mental illness severe enough to cause some level of impairment (Burns, Costello, Angold, Tweed, Stangl, Farmer, & Erkanli, 1995). Though children with emotional and behavioral disorders are found in all socioeconomic classes, all racial and ethnic groups, for some children in urban, inner city neighborhoods exposed to severe psychosocial adversity, the figure may exceed 20%. The insidious nature of poverty and other life stressors in the urban context were identified by Stern, Smith and Jang (1999) as affecting the family and parenting processes that in turn affect adolescent mental health.

This article will discuss the state of mental health for children and adolescents, particularly African American adolescents, examine barriers to effective mental health policy and programs for emotionally disturbed adolescents, and report on City Lights School, a community-based psycho-educational program that serves troubled African American adolescents and their perceptions of the program as helpful.

THE STATUS OF CHILDREN AND ADOLESCENTS MENTAL HEALTH SERVICES

A recent report released by the Surgeon General of the United States indicated that the nation faces a crisis in mental health services for children and adolescents. The report set a national agenda and outlined goals and strategies to improve services for children and adolescents with mental health problems. "Growing numbers of children are suffering needlessly because their emotional, behavioral, and developmental needs are not being met by the very institutions and systems that were created to take care of them" (Satcher, 2000). Among the children diagnosed each year with behavioral and emotional problems, fewer than one in five receives needed treatment (Burns et al., 1995; HHS NEWS, 2001).

Knitzer (1982) in *Unclaimed Children: The Failure of Public Responsibility to Children and Adolescents in Need of Mental Health Services*, a Children's Defense Fund survey of state child and adolescent mental health programs, found:

1. inadequate mental health services for this group,
2. few mental health departments with a policy focus on children and adolescents,
3. lack of coordination between those systems serving children and adolescents (child welfare, mental health, juvenile, educational),
4. lack of monitoring of children in the mental health system,
5. lack of advocacy for children with mental health needs, and
6. children underserved under existing federal programs.

This analysis produced a ringing indictment of the state of mental health services for children and adolescents in the United States. Now, almost 20 years later, the nation is again called to action to improve services for children and adolescents with mental health problems and their families. Though attempts have been made to increase access to mental health services for children and adolescents, the delivery of services remains a complex and fragmented patchwork of programs and services inaccessible to many children, especially those in poor, marginalized racial and ethnic groups.

Historically, a series of court and legislative landmarks served as the catalyst for a range of services for children with disabilities including emotional and behavioral disorders. Court decisions such as the Pennsylvania Association for Retarded Citizens v. Commonwealth (1971) and Mills v. Board of Education of the District of Columbia (1972) established the responsibility of states and localities to educate children with disabilities. In 1975, Congress enacted the Education for All Handicapped Children Act (Public Law 94-142), to support states and localities in protecting the rights of, meeting the needs of, and improving the results for children and youth (ages 3 to 21) with disabilities and their families (IDEA 25th Anniversary Website, 2000). The 1986 amendments to EHA mandated services from birth; amendments in 1990 changed the name of the EHA to Individuals with Disabilities Education Act (IDEA), and the IDEA Amendments of 1997 specified that transition planning with disabilities should begin at age 14. Theoretically, attention to children with disabilities has been continuous and IDEA has supported a number of demonstration projects around the country. However, IDEA is aimed primarily at the education system and is concerned about children with disabilities, including mental health problems, from the point of view of educating them. There is no parallel mandate to provide services to children and adolescents in the mental health system.

Despite the ongoing attention to children with disabilities and the expansion of the scope of EHA through amendments, children with mental health problems are still less likely to be identified and served appropriately. The Surgeon General of the United States, Dr. David Satcher in his Conference Report on Children's Mental Health: A National Action Agenda, proposed an initiative that identified the promotion of health in children and the treatment of mental disorders a national priority and a major public health issue. This initiative, The National Action Agenda for Children's Mental Health, took as its guiding principles a commitment to:

1. Promote the recognition of mental health as an essential part of child health;
2. Integrate family, child and youth-centered mental health services into all systems that serve children and youth;
3. Engage families and incorporate the perspectives of children and youth in the development of all mental health care planning; and
4. Develop and enhance a public-private health infrastructure to support these efforts to the fullest extent possible (Satcher, 2000; p. 5).

The adolescents who challenge the mental health system typically are not psychotic or overtly bizarre, though some with severe emotional problems may be. Rather, they are the youth who are sporadically or chronically aggressive and violent (Knitzer, 1982), or too withdrawn, have problems learning in school, or who will get into trouble with the law. Every school has its percentage of students who are failing, have difficulty relating to authority, are chronically absent, or decided to drop out of school because of unacceptable behavior and/or poor academic performance. "More than 50 percent of minority students in large cities drop out of school" (Individuals with Disabilities Education Act, 1997; p. 7). Bools, Foster, Brown and Berg (1990) found that 50% of school drop-outs have psychiatric disorders. Some of these youngsters are involved with drugs, have court records, or are in out-of-home placements. Through the school system, the mental health or juvenile justice systems, many of them have been identified as emotionally disturbed or behaviorally disordered; all are troubled and at-risk for reasons related not only to their own individual behavior and temperament, but by adverse conditions related to their environment.

Of all populations of students with disabilities in the school system, those identified as seriously emotionally disturbed have the highest dropout rates, lowest grades and academic achievement (Eber & Nelson, 1997; see also Lewis, 2000). Some research has suggested that the adverse social conditions many urban families face place children and adolescents, especially those living in inner cities, at elevated risk of mental health problems (McLoyd, 1998; Tolan & Henry, 1996). Takeuchi (2000) identifies racism as a continuous problem that creates a social environment characterized by alienation, frustration, powerlessness, stress and demoralization, all of which can adversely affect children and adolescents' mental health.

Theoretical Framework

Ecological theories of human development (Bronfenbrenner, 1986) and social work's person-in-environment perspective provide a useful framework for understanding and treating mental illness in children and adolescents. Both consider the interaction between multiple systems as determinants of positive and negative factors in physical and mental health, and social functioning (Stiffman, Hadley-Ives, Elze, Johnson, & Dore, 1999). For the most part, the exact causes of mental and behavioral disorders in childhood and adolescence are largely unknown. However, a great deal is known about the types and conditions children and adolescents suffer and the factors, particularly psychosocial ones, that place children at-risk for mental health and adjustment problems (Institute of Medicine, 1989). An ecological approach considers the transactions of the person between and among the various systems, and all aspects of the environment. Such an approach supports the outcomes projected for the adolescents in various programs–that with positive transactions and interventions, they will surmount their emotional and behavioral problems and make the transition to independence and self-sufficiency. These theories provide a contextual framework for understanding and developing preventive efforts and programmatic interventions because they seek to explain and understand the complex relationships between people and their environments (Brown & Gourdine, 1997).

BARRIERS TO MENTAL HEALTH SERVICES FOR ADOLESCENTS

Programs that set out to serve adolescents with emotional and behavior disorders face a daunting task. The nature of adolescence itself acts as a barrier to young people accessing mental health services. Adolescents are prone to engage in risky behavior (British Medical Journal, 2000) and are difficult to engage in treatment. Even though behavior problems impair their social functioning, they do not often identify their behavior as needing mental health interventions. In this respect, adolescents are no different than the general population. For despite a generally more enlightened understanding of mental illness in the 21st century, the stigma of mental illness remains a powerful and pervasive force that prevents people from acknowledging their own mental health problems (Mental Health: A Report of the Surgeon General, 1999).

The most difficult barriers to the provision of mental health services for children and adolescents, however, reside in the service delivery system itself. The responsibility for children's and adolescents' mental health is multidimensional and dispersed across multiple systems and professions: schools, primary care, the juvenile justice system, child welfare and substance abuse treatment (Satcher, 2000). Key personnel shortages among mental health professionals serving children and adolescents and under-training of other personnel working with children and adolescents have been identified as barriers to effective treatment. Funding is categorical, and funding streams are attached to individual children through Medicaid, or public programs such as those provided by schools or community mental health centers. Children and adolescent needs are increasingly defined by slots in service bureaucracies mandated to address an interlocking array of issues such as child abuse, mental health, substance abuse and delinquency and, that determined, how youth will be categorized and served (Bazemore & Terry, 1997). There is no coordinated, systematic way to provide mental health services to children and adolescents, no sharing of pools of funds to address the issue in a comprehensive way. Although great strides have been made in the treatment of adult mental illness, the capacity for diagnosing and treating childhood disorders has lagged behind. Undoubtedly, the fact that the U.S. does not have a system of health care for children and adolescents contributes to the lack of coordinated mental health services for these groups. The inability to distinguish early on the symptoms of disorders that may lead to life-long difficulties from serious, but transient dysfunction, and a desire to avoid premature labeling, often lead to under-identification of children and adolescents with mental health problems. Inner city African American adolescents with behavior problems are disproportionately more likely to be identified as criminal and tracked to the juvenile justice system (LaPoint, 2000).

CURRENT CONSIDERATIONS OF WAYS TO PROVIDE MENTAL HEALTH SERVICES TO CHILDREN AND ADOLESCENTS

In the years since the Knitzer (1982) study focused national attention on the mental health needs of children and adolescents, school districts, mental health agencies and others attempted to respond to the needs of these populations. In 1984, the National Institute of Mental Health authorized by Congress, created the Child and Adolescents Services Systems Program (CASSP). This organization provided challenge grants to states to increase collaboration among state agencies in meeting the mental health needs of children and adolescents (Knitzer, 1990). CASSP, now incarnated as the Substance Abuse and Mental Health Services Administration's (SAMHSA) Center for Mental Health Services (CMHS), has fostered a climate that led to a variety of systems change initiatives, through block grants and Knowledge, Development Application grants to states.

The traditional model of mental health services to children and adolescents prior to the 1980s consisted of office-based outpatient therapy and psychiatric residential placement. This model was handled primarily through the medical and mental health systems. Over the years, a much more complex system has evolved fueled by CASSP and others (e.g., the Robert Woods Johnson Foundation, The Annie Casey Foundation; Knitzer, 1993). Friedman (2000) advocates for a systems of care approach that he defined as "a comprehensive spectrum of mental health and other necessary services that are organized into a coordinated network to meet the multiple and changing needs of children and adolescents with severe emotional disturbances and their families" (p. 40). The Surgeon General, Dr. Satcher, proposes that one way to respond to children's mental health needs is to "move the country toward a community health system that balances health promotion, disease prevention, early detection and offers universal access to care" (Satcher, 2000 p. 14). Another evidenced-based approach supported by research funds from the National Institute of Mental Health (NIMH) is Multisystemic Therapy (MST). MST has been found effective for interventions with youth across the service systems. It is a strengths perspective home-based model of therapy that focuses on changing how youths function in their natural settings–at home, in school, and in their neighborhoods (Henggeler, Schoenwald, Borduin, Mann, & Cone, 1998), and is designed to strengthen the ability of parents or caretakers to raise children who have complex problems.

Baenen, Stephens, and Glenwick (1986) cite the educational, legal, and social policy support for the role of psycho-educational day school programs in fulfilling the objectives of special services to behavior-disordered children. Gall, Pagano, Desmond, Perrin, and Murphy (2001) examined the potential of school-based health centers to improve the recognition and treatment of adolescents' mental health problems. Although school-based health centers have substantial potential to improve the recognition and treatment of adolescents' mental health problems, there is a place in the continuum of interventions for separate community day treatment programs. These programs can serve that portion of the school population where the severity of the behavior compromises the adolescents' ability to remain in the regular school setting but does not qualify them for residential treatment. African American adolescents, especially males, are more likely to be identified as behavior problems, suspended, and barred from school until they drop out and drift to the juvenile justice system where it is even less likely they will be treated for mental health problems. The model of community-based psychoeducation day treatment programs can be an effective intervention with this population of youth if, in addition to treatment, the programs embrace the strengths perspective advocated by Bazemore and Terry (1997) that considers youth as resources to the community and capable of mastering a competency-based approach to academic and vocational habilitation.

CITY LIGHTS SCHOOL: A MODEL PROGRAM SERVING URBAN AFRICAN AMERICAN ADOLESCENTS

City Lights School, Inc., is a community-based private psycho-educational day school treatment program in Washington, D. C. founded in 1982 with the support of the Children's Defense Fund. The program was a direct response to the CDF-sponsored 1982 survey by Knitzer, which indicated a dearth of programs serving emotionally and behaviorally disordered children and adolescents. City Lights is committed to providing quality educational, clinical and vocational services to some of the most difficult youth in the District of Columbia and provides a community alternative to more restrictive placements in residential psychiatric facilities.

City Lights School provides a program to educate troubled adolescents in a therapeutic milieu where the education program itself becomes one of the tools for treatment. The education and clinical components of the program work together to establish a consistent, coherent, treatment plan for youth whose lives in the past have been fragmented and unpredictable (Tolmach, 1985). City Lights School features a multidisciplinary treatment approach involving mental health and special education professionals, low teacher-pupil ratios, services to the youths' families, advocacy among systems and a goal of reintegration into the educational or vocational mainstream. In addition to an academic curriculum that meets the District of Columbia Public School's (DCPS) criteria for high school graduation, students receive individual and group therapy, art therapy, social living skills, a daily class meeting, weekly community meetings, anger management, and peer mediation training. In addition, City Lights boasts a new state-of-the-art culinary program, an industrial arts building and curriculum to strengthen the vocational component of the special education/treatment program, and a structured after-school program to provide a safe haven for the youth without a community network of social supports. For those adolescents unable to go on to technical school or college, it provides the level of support needed to help seriously emotionally disordered adolescents transition to jobs. The program employs a behavior modification contingency system based on points for appropriate behavior, peer mediation training, and intensive outreach to the other systems involved with the students–the family, group homes, child welfare, probation officers, etc.

City Lights is used here as an example of a program whose history reflects the uncertain and uncoordinated funding for mental health services for adolescents and highlights the dilemma sometimes faced when serving this population. When the program was started almost 20 years ago with private funds, there was no one place to go to request funds or to access the population of adolescents needing mental health services. City Lights, through private funding, provided unsolicited free slots to the various systems serving adolescents to educate the personnel in various systems to the viability of serving seriously emotionally disturbed adolescents in a community-based day treatment program. The first system to utilize City Lights and eventually fund placements for emotionally disturbed adolescents was the Commission on Mental Health Services (CMHS), followed by the child welfare system (Commission on Social Services, CSS) under court order to bring children back from residential placements in other states to a less restrictive placement in their community. The juvenile justice system through the D.C. Superior Court and later the Youth Services Administration (YSA) sought to utilize portions of the program for adjudicated youth (for GED preparation, job placement, transition back to the community from a juvenile facility, etc.), but would not fund the cost of the program that covered mental health even though the adolescents referred from YSA had moderate to severe emotional and behavioral disorders.

City Lights utilized a program within a program model to serve the adjudicated youth apart from its day treatment program, nevertheless, CMHS and CSS discontinued placing children at City Lights because these systems did not want youth they were responsible for in the same environment with youth from the juvenile justice system. The school system used the placement sporadically, usually encouraged by lawyers in the special education hearing process for special youth from the juvenile justice system.

Despite the efforts of City Lights to house three programs in its building and provide services related to funding streams, the funding as well as the referral sources' perception of the needs of the adolescents they served were different. Lack of a predictable funding source and the agency absorbing much of the cost of mental health services to court-referred youth led City Lights to revamp its program in line with the needs of the public school system. Currently, DCPS refers the majority of the adolescents served at City Lights School. The program again faces a challenge from the proliferation of charter schools in Washington, D. C. And the school is moving to establish a special education charter school serving younger children. A snapshot of the youth served by the program was developed from data collected for *City Lights School: Their Second Last Chance*, a review of the program over the last 12 years.

Description of Youth Served

The adolescents who attend City Lights are those marginalized by the effects of myriad negative social indicators–poverty, drugs, violence, school failure, dysfunctional families–and are those that are generally too disturbed for the regular classroom school setting. A profile of the students at three points in the history of City Lights shows that males have consistently comprised a larger percentage of the population, that 60% or more of the adolescents in the program had a history of juvenile offenses even though only one year, 1992, represented an influx of adolescents from the juvenile justice system. The average length of stay in the program has also increased from 9.0 months in 1992 to 15.5 months in 2000 (see Table 1).

Other indications of the type of students served by City Lights is found in the psychiatric diagnoses of the students and prior placements in more restrictive settings. Sixty-one percent of the students in 2000 are diagnosed with behavior disorders compared to 38% in 1989. The difference could well reflect better record keeping or the requirement of diagnosis at admission. Twenty percent of the students had a placement in a residential treatment facility (see Table 2).

For the most part, the students served by City Lights are not the kind of students whose mental health and educational problems would be served well in special education classrooms within the school setting. The issues that must be addressed for the students include not only their own mental health issues but concern and attention to their lives in the community. It is clear from the experience of the City Lights School in its various incarnations over the past almost 20 years, that children with serious behavior problems can be reached through programs geared to meet their needs. A survey of the students in the 2000 school year indicated that 86% felt they had a positive relationship with the staff. Eighty percent felt they could trust the staff, a significant outcome for a group of students who often feel they have no one in their lives they can trust.

TABLE 1. Profile of Students

Demographics	1989	1992	2000*
Average age at admission	17.9	16.7	15.9
Average months in program	9.9	9.0	15.5 months
Males	65%	74%	7%
Females	35%	26%	30%
Students in program < = six months	33%	38%	19%
Students in program > = one year	67%	62%	81%
African Americans	98%	99%	97%
Latinos	2%	1%	3%
History of juvenile offense	60%	82%	61%

From City Lights School: Their Last Second Chance (2000). Printed with permission.
*N = 35

TABLE 2. Clinical Characteristics

Diagnosis	1989	1992	2000*
Psychosis	5%	2%	4%
Behavior Disorder	38%	54%	61%
Depressive Mood/Disorder	37%	34%	34%
Anxiety Disorder	N/A	N/A	7%
Learning Disorder	N/A	N/A	19%
Mild Mental Retardation/MR	N/A	N/A	15%
Substance Use (self-reported)	N/A	58%	61%
Diagnosed as Substance Abusers	N/A	N/A	11%
Prior placement in Residential Treatment	N/A	N/A	20%
Prior placement in a Psychiatric Hospital	N/A	12%	24%

City Lights School: Their Last Second Chance. Printed with permission.
*N = 35

One thing is clear, however, there is no quick fix for helping youngsters who are seriously emotionally and/or behaviorally disordered. A follow-up survey by City Lights of a convenience sample of 25 of 158 students who exited the program between 1996 and 1999, those students who received a high school diploma or certificate of attainment or who were in school or vocational training at the time of the survey, were associated with the program the longest on average, 24.6 months and 12.7 months respectively. Those students found to be incarcerated at the time of follow-up were associated with the program an average of 3.3 months.

DISCUSSION

Model programs like City Lights are just one piece of the puzzle to providing mental health services to troubled inner-city adolescents. Children with mental health problems have complex and multiple needs. The service delivery system must have a continuum of services including prevention and early identification to adequately address the mental health needs of children and adolescents. The majority of mental health services delivered to children and youth are not delivered in the formal mental health service system (Costello, Burns, Angold, & Leaf, 1993). Therefore, a fiscal infrastructure forged through cross-systems collaboration is needed to ensure that children and adolescents with mental health disabilities are served across the developmental spectrum. IDEA, through its mandates to serve all children with disabilities including behaviorally and emotionally disturbed adolescents, has broadened the scope of services to severely emotionally disturbed children and youth. Nevertheless, the collaboration among various agencies has done little to increase the reality of shared resources. The literature in special education is replete with innovative models for serving emotionally disturbed children and adolescents in the school system. Seemingly absent from the discussion is the role of the community mental health system. The once promising conceptualization of the role of community mental health centers in the prevention of mental illness appears all but abandoned. This author was involved in a community mental health center's primary prevention outreach programs of the early 1980s at Chesterfield Community Mental Health Center that provided consultation to nursery schools, groups for anger management, children of divorce and problem-solving skills in the public school system, and parent education groups in libraries and public health waiting rooms. This is evidence that community mental health centers through primary prevention programs could work with other systems (especially schools) around early identification and intervention. The question, of course, then and now is who will pay for these kinds of interventions. Schools can and should play an important role in the provision of services and funding for programs for children and adolescents with mental health disabilities. However, school systems alone can not carry the responsibility. There is too much of a cumulative knowledge base and evidenced-based practice interventions in other systems, as well as the differential needs of emotionally and behaviorally disordered children and adolescents themselves, for one system to carry the responsibility for service provision to this population.

The inequity in funding for schools is already an issue manifest in an ongoing national discussion of differential resources, deteriorating physical facilities and quality of education. The poorest school districts are also likely to have the larger percentage of children needing mental health services given the link between poor environmental conditions and negative mental health consequences. Will only those school districts able to write grants and develop programs have the capacity to provide mental health services to their students? School systems are concerned about the overall population of students needing an education and are, therefore, worried about the increasing expenditures from their budgets for special education. The complexity of the issues around provision of mental health services to children and adolescents makes it impossible to think of a single-system solution. There will necessarily be multiple solutions requiring systemic collaboration from the national to the local levels and across professional domains.

IMPLICATION FOR SOCIAL WORK PRACTICE

Social workers are in a unique position to contribute to shaping the system of services for children with mental health needs. Social workers practice across the human service delivery system spectrum. They are heavily represented in practice in the mental health system and increasing in numbers in school systems. LaPointe (2000) noted that school systems need to revisit the role social workers and other professionals can play in developing mental health prevention and treatment programs. Though school social work is not new, it is only in recent years that some school districts have included social workers as a part of their staffs. Now it is important for school administrators to know how to use their expertise. Social workers have always embraced a holistic approach to intervention and understand the need for an integrated system of mental health care for children and adolescents. While social workers are frontline workers in a large part of the work force in child welfare and community mental health centers, and are represented in the work force of the school and juvenile justice systems, they are not often in positions of leadership at the level where policy is developed. With a model of practice that emphasizes a systemic approach to providing interventions, it is clear that social workers have much to contribute to any national or local efforts aimed at developing an integrated system of mental health services for children and adolescents.

REFERENCES

Bazemore, G. & Terry, W. C. (1997). Developing delinquent youths: A reintegrative model for rehabilitation and a new role for the juvenile justice system. *Child Welfare, 76* (5), 665-715.

Bools, C., Foster, J., Brown, I., & Berg, I. (1990). The identification of psychiatric disorders in children who fail to attend school: A cluster analysis of a non-clinical population. *Psychological Medicine, 20,* 171-181.

British Medical Journal (2000). Adolescent mental health and risky sexual behavior (Editorial). *British Medical Journal, 321* (7256), 251-252.

Brofenbrenner, U. (1986). Ecology of the family as a context for human development: Research perspectives. *Developmental Psychology, 22,* 723-742.

Brown, A. & Gourdine, R. (1998). Teenage black girls and violence: Coming of age in an urban environment. *Journal of Human Behavior in the Social Environment, 1* (2/3), 105-124.

Burns, B. J., Costello, E. J., Angold, A., Tweed, D., Stangl, D., Farmer, E. M. Z. & Erkanli, A. (1995). Data watch: Children's mental health service use across service sectors. *Health Affair, 14* (3), 147-159.

Costello, J., Burns, B., Angold, A., & Leaf, P. (1993). How can epidemiology improve mental health services for children and adolescents. *Journal of the American Academy of Child and Adolescent Psychiatry, 32* (6), 1106-1114.

Davis, Owen (2000). *Their last second chance: The story of City Lights School.* Washington, DC: City Lights School, Inc.

Eber, L. E. & Nelson, M. (1997). School-based wraparound planning: Integrating services for students with emotional and behavioral needs. *American Journal of Orthopsychiatry, 67*(3), 385-394.

Friedman, R., Katz-Leavy, J., Manderschied, R., & Sondheimer, D. (1996). Prevalence of serious emotional disturbance among children and adolescents. In R. W. Manderchied & A. Sonnerchein (Eds.), *Mental health, United States, 1996: SAMHSA Mental health services* (Chapter 6). <http://www.nccbh.org/html/learn/books/SAMHSA-toc.htm>.

Friedman, R. M. (2000). Panel Discussion: Systems of care: Financing and organizing service systems. *Proceedings based on the Surgeon General's Conference on Children's Mental Health: Developing a National Action Agenda* (p. 40-41). U. S. Department of Health and Human Services, The Virtual Office of the Surgeon General, <http://www. surgeongeneral. gov/cmh/childreport.htm>.

Gall, G., Pagano, M. E., Desmond, M. S., Perrin, J. M., & Murphy, J. M. (2000). Utility of psychosocial screening at a school-based health center. *Journal of School Health, 70* (7), 292-298.

Henggeler, S. W., Schoenwald, S. K., & Borduin, C. M. (1998). *Multisystemic treatment of antisocial behavior in children and adolescents.* New York: Guilford Press.

Individual with Disabilities Education Act 25th Anniversary Website–Lesson 1: History. <http://www.ed.gov/offices/OSERS/IDEA25th/Lesson_History.html>.

Individual with Disabilities Education Act, Amendments of 1997, 20 U.S.C. 1400 *et seq.*

Institute of Medicine (1989). *Research on children and adolescents with mental, behavioral and developmental disorders: Mobilizing a national initiative.* Washington, DC: National Academy Press.

Kelleher, K. J. & Wolraich, M. L. (1996). Diagnosing psychosocial problems. *Pediatrics, 97*, 899-901.

Knitzer, J. (1982). Unclaimed children: The failure of public responsibility to children and adolescents in need of mental health services. Washington, DC: The Children's Defense Fund.

Knitzer, J. (1993). Children's mental health policy: Challenging the future. *Journal of Emotional and Behavioral Disorders, 1* (1), 8-17. Retrieved June 7, 2001 from Academic Search Elite database.

LaPoint, V. (2000). Juvenile justice and identification of mental health needs. (Discussant) *Proceedings based on the Surgeon General's Conference on Children's Mental Health: Developing a National Action Agenda* (pp. 25-26). U. S. Department of Health and Human Services, The Virtual Office of the Surgeon General. <http:// www.surgeongeneral.gov/cmh/childreport.htm>.

Lewis, T. (2000). Panel Discussion: State of the evidence on treatments, services, systems of care, and financing. *Proceedings based on the Surgeon General's Conference on Children's Mental Health: Developing a National Action Agenda* (pp. 33-34). U. S. Department of Health and Human Services, The Virtual Office of the Surgeon General. <http://www.surgeongeneral.gov/cmh/childreport.htm>.

McLoyd, V. C. (1998). Socioeconomic disadvantage and child development. *American Psychologist, 53*, 185-204.

Satcher, D. (2000). Report of the Surgeon General's Conference on Children's Mental Health: A National Action Agenda. U. S. Department of Health and Human Services, The Virtual Office of the Surgeon General. <http://www.surgeongeneral. gov/cmh/childreport.htm>.

Stern, S. B., Smith, C. A., & Jang, S. J. (1999). Urban families and adolescent mental health. *Social Work Research, 23* (1), 15-27.

Stiffman, A. R., Hadley-Ives, E. Eize, D. Johnson, S. & Dore, P. (1999). Impact of environment on adolescent mental health and behavior: Structural equation modeling. *American Journal of Orthopsychiatry, 69* (1), 73-86.

Surgeon General Releases a National Action Agenda on Children's Mental Health (2001, January 3). *HHS NEWS*, p. 1. U. S. Department of Health and Human Services, The Virtual Office of the Surgeon General: <http://www.surgeongeneral. gov/todo...sreleases/ pressreleasechildren. htm>.

Takeuchi, D. T. (2000). Panel Discussion: Diversity: Access, barriers, and quality. *Proceedings based on the Surgeon General's Conference on Children's Mental Health: Developing a National Action Agenda* (p. 27). U. S. Department of Health and Human Services, The Virtual Office of the Surgeon General. <http://www.surgeongeneral.gov/cmh/childreport.htm>.

Tolan, P. H. & Henry, D. (1996). Patterns of psychopathology among urban-poor children: Co-morbidity and aggression effects. *Journal of Consulting and Clinical Psychology, 64*, 1094-1099.

Tolmach, J. There ain't nobody on my side: A new day treatment program for Black urban youth. *Journal of Clinical Child Psychology, 14* (3), 216-219.

U.S. Congress (1997). Individuals with Developmental Disabilities Act.

U.S. Department of Health and Human Services (1999). *Mental Health: A Report of the Surgeon General–Executive Summary*. Rockville, MD: U.S. Department of Health and Human Services, Substance Abuse and Mental Health Services Administration, Center for Mental Health Services, National Institutes of Health, National Institute of Mental Health. <http:\\www.surgeon general gov/library/mentalhealth/ summary.html>.

100% Access, Zero Health Disparities, and GIS: An Improved Methodology for Designating Health Professions Shortage Areas

Paul D. Juarez, PhD
Paul L. Robinson, PhD
Patricia Matthews-Juarez, PhD

SUMMARY. The (Health Professions Shortage Areas) HPSA designation process was developed as a mechanism to identify primary care shortage areas eligible for participation in specific federally funded programs including a 10% Medicare supplement, the National Health Service Corps, and health professions training programs. The purpose of this paper was to explore the utility of Geographic Information Systems (GIS) technology as an improved methodology for obtaining HPSA designation status for geographic areas. Results showed that GIS identified 24 Medical Services Study Areas (rational planning areas) in Los An-

Paul D. Juarez is affiliated with White Memorial Medical Center, Family Practice Residency Program, Los Angeles, CA.

Paul L. Robinson is affiliated with Charles R. Drew University, Los Angeles, CA.

Patricia Matthews-Juarez is affiliated with Charles R. Drew University, Los Angeles, CA.

[Haworth co-indexing entry note]: "100% Access, Zero Health Disparities, and GIS: An Improved Methodology for Designating Health Professions Shortage Areas." Juarez, Paul D., Robinson, Paul L. and Patricia Matthews-Juarez. Co-published simultaneously in *Journal of Health & Social Policy* (The Haworth Press, Inc.) Vol. 16, No. 1/2, 2002, pp. 155-167; and: *Disability and the Black Community* (ed: Sheila D. Miller) The Haworth Press, Inc., 2002, pp. 155-167. Single or multiple copies of this article are available for a fee from The Haworth Document Delivery Service [1-800-HAWORTH, 9:00 a.m. - 5:00 p.m. (EST). E-mail address: docdelivery@haworthpress.com].

geles County that met the minimum 3500:1 population-to-primary-care physician ratio for geographic area HPSA designation compared to only three that currently are identified. Authors concluded that restructuring of the state/county responsibilities for HPSA designation is long overdue and that use of GIS as a required methodology would help ensure that all areas in any state that meet the intent of federal legislation are included. *[Article copies available for a fee from The Haworth Document Delivery Service: 1-800-HAWORTH. E-mail address: <docdelivery@haworthpress.com> Website: <http:// www.HaworthPress.com> © 2002 by The Haworth Press, Inc. All rights reserved.]*

KEYWORDS. GIS, medically underserved, federal HPSA designation

Disparities of health status among residents of inner city and rural areas in the United States, especially among ethnic minority groups, in large part are attributed to unequal access to primary health care (American Academy of Pediatrics, 1981; McNutt, 1981; Smeloff, Burnett, & Kelzer, 1981; USDHHS, 1981; Blendon, Aiken, Freeman, & Corey, 1989; Council on Graduate Medical Education, 1992, 1996, 1998). The inequitable geographic distribution of primary care practitioners (PPP) is a leading cause of the lack of access (USDHEW, 1976; U.S. GAO, 1978a, 1978b; Cornelius, 1983, 1993). While recognition of geographic maldistribution of physicians was recognized as far back as 1933 (Lee & Jones, 1933), it was not until 1967 that the Report of National Advisory Commission on Health Manpower declared a national shortage of physicians (Miller, 1967). Since that time, a number of federal health policy initiatives have been undertaken to address the persistent problem of unequal health care access by supporting efforts to create incentives for physicians to practice in underserved areas. Laws passed to address health care shortages include the Critical Health Manpower Shortage Area Act (P.L. No. 91-623), the Health Manpower Shortage Areas Act (P.L. No. 94-484), and the Health Professions Educational Assistance Act of 1976.

Despite numerous reports of an increasing surplus of both sub-specialists and primary care physicians in recent years (Office of the President, 1999), there continues to exist physician shortage areas in both inner city and rural areas (COGME, 1998). To address these persistent disparities, the Bureau of Primary Health Care (BPHC) initiated a national campaign in 1998, for "100% Access and Zero Health Disparities." The identified mission of the campaign was to enroll and support community leaders in setting and achieving clear, measurable goals for attaining 100% access to health care and eliminating disparities based on race, ethnicity, gender, age, sexual preference, or income. Yet, despite these various efforts, significant disparities continue to exist in both health access and outcomes among inner city and rural populations, a majority of the nation's medically underserved (Office of the President, 1999).

The Health Professions Shortage Areas (HPSA) designation process was developed as a policy to identify primary care shortage areas eligible for participation in certain federally funded programs. Under the law, three categories of HPSA designations are identified:

1. urban and rural geographic areas,
2. population groups, and
3. facilities with shortages of health professionals.

Criteria for designating HPSAs are:

1. the geographic area involved is rational for the delivery of health services;
2. the population-to-clinician ratio representing shortage is exceeded within the area; and
3. resources in contiguous areas are overutilized, excessively distant, or otherwise inaccessible (42 CFR Part 5, 1980, as amended).

The designation process includes capturing and analyzing local demographic and economic information for specific geographic areas; identifying the numbers of primary care providers and the amount of time they practice in the area; surveying the community under consideration; interviewing primary care physicians, hospital administrators, community leaders, etc., in the identified community; and submitting the required supporting documentation for the application of the area, population, or facility to be designated. This application process is cumbersome, time intensive, and expensive. The result of this complex and difficult process is lost opportunities to increase access to primary health care services to vulnerable and disadvantaged communities because many areas, populations, and facilities that are eligible to receive HPSA designation fail to get identified and reviewed.

The purpose of this paper is to explore the utility of Geographic Information Systems (GIS) technology as an improved methodology for obtaining HPSA designation status for geographic areas, in order to increase the incentives to attract more primary care physicians to underserved areas and promote the national goals of 100% Access and Zero Health Disparities. A comparison of the HPSA designations identified in the Federal Register for Los Angeles County dated September 15, 2000 with those that can be demonstrated to have met federal criteria for HPSA designation using GIS is presented as an example of the utility of GIS technology. Recommendations and policy implications are offered.

DESCRIPTION OF THE APPLICATION PROCESS
FOR HPSA DESIGNATION

Section 332 of the Public Health Services Act, 42 U.S.C. 254e gives the Secretary of the Department of Health and Human Services the authority to designate Health Professions Shortage Areas (HPSAs) based on criteria established in 1980 final regulations (42 CFR Part 5) and Health Resources and Services Administration's (HRSA) Bureau of Primary Health Care (BPHC), and the Division of Shortage Designation the direct responsibility for designating and updating HPSAs. The process begins with the submission of an application requesting a HPSA designation to the Bureau of Primary Health Care (BPHC) and/or the appropriate State Health Planning and Development Agency (SHPDA) or a unit of the State Health Department by interested organizations and individuals. An applicant must respond to the federal criteria and demonstrate that the requested area is a rational area. Once the rational area has been determined, the applicant must calculate the population using the federal formula to adjust for expected number of patient visits. After the calculations have been completed, the applicant must count and survey the primary care physicians practicing in the area under study. Criteria are also presented for determining an unusually high need for primary medical services, an insufficient capacity of existing primary care providers, consideration of primary care capacity in contiguous areas, and the degree of primary care physician shortage.

Rational area. The initial step in requesting a HPSA designation for a geographic area is to demonstrate that the area is rational for the delivery of primary care services. The criteria can be met by demonstrating that:

1. the population centers are within 30 minutes travel time of each other,
2. the topography, market or transportation patterns limit access to PCPs in contiguous areas, and
3. the established neighborhoods and communities display a strong self-identity.

Travel time is calculated on a distance of 30 minutes or less based on type of roadway. For rural areas, the general rule is 20 miles with primary roads under normal conditions; 15 miles in mountainous terrain or in areas where only secondary roads are available; and 25 miles in flat terrain or in areas connected by interstate highways. For urban areas, travel time is calculated based on 30 minutes on public transportation. Travel distance criteria are easily addressed using linear network analysis, a well-established function of commercial GIS products, such as ESRI's *Network Analyst.* Calculation of travel areas using GIS can account for not only distances, but also more complex factors such as speed limit, traffic density, and turning times.

Population count. The second step of the HPSA designation process is to calculate the population in a rational area, adjusting for age and gender, based on expected number of primary care visits for twelve, age X gender groups. To calculate expected numbers of primary care visits for each of the twelve age X gender groups, national data, available through the Federal Register and the Bureau of Primary Health Care/HRSA, are used and multiplied by the actual population for the same age X gender cohort in the rational area. The total expected visit rate is obtained by multiplying each of the 12 expected visit rates by the total number of permanent residents in the area for each age X gender cohort, summing them, and dividing the grand total by 5.1, the total U.S. average per capita visit rate. The result is the total population count for the area adjusted for expected primary care visits. Where warranted, further adjustments to the population count are to be made to account for the effects of transient populations, including tourists, migratory workers and their families, and seasonal residents.

Primary care practitioners count. The third step is to calculate the number of full-time equivalent (FTE), non-federal, primary care doctors of medicine and osteopathy who provide direct patient care in outpatient clinics in the target geographic area. For this purpose, primary care practitioners (PCP) are identified as General Practice physicians and those that completed residency training in Family Practice, General Internal Medicine, Pediatrics, and OB/GYN. Excluded from the PCP count are primary care physicians who are engaged full-time in research, administration and teaching, graduates of foreign medical schools who are not citizens or lawful permanent U.S. residents, physicians who practice exclusively in inpatient care, and physicians whose Medicare or Medicaid licenses have been suspended for a period of 18 months or more. The PCP count is to be adjusted further for interns and residents, semi-retired physicians who operate a reduced practice or provide patient care in an area less than full-time, and graduates of foreign medical schools who are citizens or lawful permanent residents of the United States but do not have unrestricted licenses to practice. In addition, allowances may be made for physicians located within an area who are not accessible to the population.

Determination of unusually high needs for primary medical services. An area will be considered as having unusually high needs for primary health care services if any one of the following three criteria is met:

1. the area has more than 100 births per year per 1,000 women ages 15-44;
2. the area has more than 20 infant deaths per 1,000 women ages 15-44; or
3. more than 20% of the population has an income below the poverty level.

Determination of insufficient capacity of existing primary care providers.
An area's PCP capacity is determined insufficient when at least two of the following criteria are met:

1. FTE primary care physicians serving the area provide greater than 8,000 office or outpatient visits per year;
2. waiting time for appointments for routine medical services is more than seven days for established patients and 14 days for new patients;
3. average waiting time in primary care provider offices is greater than one hour where patients have appointments or two hours where patients are treated on a walk-in basis;
4. there is evidence of excessive patient use of emergency rooms for routine care;
5. two thirds or more of the area's PCPs do not accept new patients; or
6. the average utilization of health services by the population of the area is less than 2.0 visits per year.

Contiguous areas. To receive a HPSA designation, PCP services in areas contiguous to the target area need to be demonstrated as excessively distant, overutilized or inaccessible to the population. Inaccessibility in contiguous areas can be demonstrated by any one of the three following criteria:

1. PCPs in the contiguous area are more than 30 minutes travel time from the population center(s) of the area being considered for HPSA designation;
2. the population to PCP ratio in the contiguous area must be in excess of 2,000:1; or
3. PCPs in the contiguous areas are inaccessible due to significant differences between the socioeconomic status of the area under consideration or when the poverty rate of the contiguous area is greater than 20%.

Determination of degree of shortage. Designated areas are assigned to a degree of shortage group based upon the ratio of population to full-time equivalent PCP and whether or not unusually high needs are indicated.

METHODOLOGY

Geographic Information Systems technology makes it possible to standardize the steps involved in the HPSA designation application process, including documenting the rational area, population count, primary care practitioner count, determination of unusually high needs for primary medical services, contiguous areas, and degree of shortage. GIS uses a relational database that incorporates digital geography information and can be used to identify sub-populations that cluster by demographics, health status, and socioeconomic background to more effectively target underserved populations. According to Wieczorek (1998) the main functions of GIS are:

1. to geo-code data by providing a spatial reference (x,y coordinates) based on address,
2. to combine the contents of multiple maps or data layers by overlaying them in a single operation (i.e., a relational data base),
3. to reclassify data based on queries, and
4. to measure distance, adjacency and connectivity between geographical entities (p. 2).

Important features of a GIS include: geo-coding-address matching, layering-linking of data bases, reclassification, distance and adjacency function, buffer function, neighborhood functions and spatial cluster analyses. A more comprehensive overview of these functions is presented in his unpublished paper "Using Geographic Information Systems for Small Area Analysis" (Wieczorek, 1998). The mapping and address matching features of a GIS are important features that lend it to being an ideal technology for the HPSA designation process. Address mapping is synonymous with the term "geo-coding" and is the main source of spatial data for small area demographic social and economic analysis (Drummonds, 1995).

Data files used included 2000 U.S. Census Tiger street address files, 1990 TIGER census tract boundary files for Los Angeles County and 1990 Census data by census tract (Department of Commerce, 1990). While 2000 U.S. Census data are beginning to be released, a breakdown by age and gender by census tract is not yet available.

GIS was used in this study to examine 87 MSSAs in Los Angeles County to demonstrate its utility as a methodology for identifying geographic areas that meet federal HPSA designation criteria. MSSAs are geographical areas, established in 1976 by the California Office of Statewide Health Planning and Development (OSHPD), to identify priority urban and rural areas of unmet need for family physicians for the purpose of carrying out the mandate of the Song-Brown Family Practice Act. An agreement was reached with HRSA in 1995 to use MSSAs as the basis for establishing rational areas for all subsequent HPSA designation requests in the State of California (Burnett, 2001). A list of the 87 Medical Service Study Areas (MSSA) and their boundary files used to identify Rational Areas in Los Angeles County was obtained from the California Office of Statewide Health Planning and Development (OSHPD).

GIS was used to calculate the population count by age, gender, and race/ethnicity for MSSAs. Population counts were then adjusted based on expected number of visits by age and gender, summed, and divided by 5.1 to obtain an adjusted population for each MSSA in the County of Los Angeles. ArcView

GIS software was used to attach the state MSSA data files to the 1990 GIS boundary file so that the HPSA designation analysis could be conducted with each MSSA serving as a rational area. The *57,000 Physicians and Surgeons Directory* (infoUSA, 2001) was used to identify primary care physicians' offices in Los Angeles County by address and specialty. Primary care physicians were identified as Family Practice, General Pediatrics, OB/GYN, General Internal Medicine, and General Practice. Of 1,381 Family Physicians identified from the database as practicing in Los Angeles County, 28 also identified as General Practice, 71 as Internal Medicine, 17 as OB/GYN, 19 as Pediatrics, and 46 as others. Physicians who were identified as having another specialty were not included on the list of Family Physicians. After eliminating those who identified with another specialty, a total of 1,200 Family Physicians remained. Using the same process, a total of 1,156 Pediatricians, 918 OB/GYN, 641 General Practice, and 2,057 Internal Medicine physicians were identified.

RESULTS

Batch matching of the physician practice database yielded an 88.3% (5,034 of 5,698) match rate. Because of this high accuracy rate, no further efforts were undertaken to interactively rematch addresses. Analysis of land area covered by the three geographic areas in Los Angeles County currently designated as HPSAs by the Division of Shortage Designation, BHPR/HRSA as of July 31, 2000 (Federal Register, Vol. 65, No. 180, Friday, September 15, 2000) shows that approximately 150 square miles, or 3.7% of the land area of Los Angeles County currently has a geographic area HPSA designation. (See Figure 1.)

According to current BPHC HPSA designations, 195,741 individuals (1990 U.S. Census) live in areas with a geographic area HPSA designation in Los Angeles County. Persons residing (1990 U.S. Census) in the three currently designated geographic area HPSAs comprise 2.2% of the total population of Los Angeles County; 2.2% of males and 2.2% of females; and 4.3% of Blacks, 4.2% of Latinos, and 1.1% of Whites.

In contrast, when GIS was used to identify HPSA geographic areas that meet the 3500:1 population to PPP ratio, 24 MSSAs were identified. The areas identified as meeting federal criteria for HPSA designation using GIS accounted for 1,651 square miles, or 40% of the area of Los Angeles County (see Figure 2). The total population within these combined areas is 2,373,758 (1990 U.S. Census), 1,798,558 greater than a methodology that does not employ GIS. Taken together, persons residing in GIS identified geographic area HPSAs comprise 26.7% of the total population of Los Angeles County; 26.7%

FIGURE 1. Current Areas with Geographic Area and Population HPSA Designations: Los Angeles County, July 31, 2000

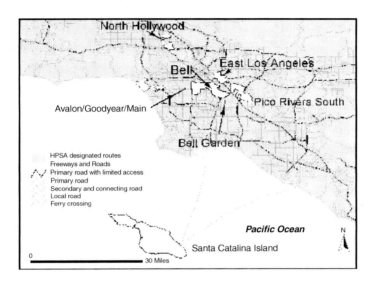

of males and 26.7% of females; and 49% of Blacks, 32% of Latinos, and 21% of Whites.

DISCUSSION

The current process for designating primary care medically underserved areas as HPSAs is haphazard and cumbersome, at best. Despite the advantages of being designated a HPSA, there are no requirements that mandate or facilitate applications for HPSA designation. In states and/or localities in which Health Departments do not undertake the task of applying for HPSA designation for qualified areas, this responsibility is left to the willingness and determination of local agencies and individuals to undertake. The application is time consuming and assumes access to information that may or may not be readily available. This HPSA designation process involves various stages, most of which can be accomplished with the manipulation of large databases. Without the capacity to manipulate large databases, however, the task of mapping becomes a manual, time intensive one. A new methodology for substantiating areas, populations, and facilities is very much needed.

FIGURE 2. GIS Derived Areas that Meet Federal Geographic Area HPSA Criteria: Los Angeles County (1990 U.S. Census)

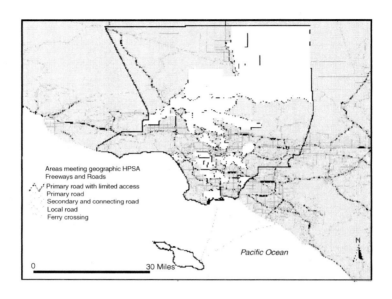

Despite BPHC's goal of 100% Access and Zero Health Disparities, many primary care underserved areas, populations, and facilities that are eligible based on federal criteria, never receive a HPSA designation, primarily because no one submits the paperwork. This is a seriously flawed process that results in some of the most underserved populations not receiving HPSA designation and prevents deserving communities from accessing the benefits that would otherwise be made available to them. In addition to the three currently identified geographic areas HPSAs in Los Angeles County, six additional areas have population HPSA designations. Of the nine total currently designated geographic area and population HPSAs in Los Angeles County, only two are among the top 12 GIS identified geographic area and population HPSAs. Ten of the top 12 most medically underserved areas in Los Angeles County currently do not have either a geographic area or population HPSA designation.

Social policy implications. Results of this paper suggest that GIS offers a greatly improved methodology for undertaking the HPSA designation process. Clearly, the existing system is incomplete and, as in the case of Los Angeles County, resulted in 10 of 12 of the poorest and most underserved areas being left off of the HPSA designation list. Results from a policy perspective suggest a need to dramatically alter the HPSA designation process to fulfill legislative intent. We are recommending that the application process for HPSA designation be the total responsibility of the state to ensure that all communities eligible to receive a HPSA designation are designated. We further recommend that the HPSA designation process be implemented in two phases. The first part of the application process should entail updating the methodology for data gathering and collection. As demonstrated by this paper, states should adopt a methodology that employs GIS. Use of GIS technology would enhance efficiency and save time and money for states, local government, and community groups and individuals that currently are left to their own resources to apply for HPSA designations for geographic areas and populations. The second phase of the HPSA designation process would involve the community under study for designation. Community residents could be involved in street verification of the sites, verification of the medical need, and commenting on PCP accessibility and data analyses. This verification process by communities would be essential to ensure that analyses capture local community nuances that might otherwise be missed.

Limitations. These analyses present an initial effort to use GIS as a methodology to identify areas eligible for geographic area HPSA designation and as such, the results should be considered preliminary. There remain a number of limiting factors that need to be studied further to perfect this methodology.

Use of the 1990 U.S. Census is a limitation of this paper. Population shifts in some communities between the 1990 and 2000 Census could affect the HPSA designation status of some MSSAs. Given that the population of Los Angeles County grew by 656,174 between 1990 and 2000, it is likely that these population to PCP ratios are underestimates that will increase after adjustments for population growth are made.

Primary care physicians were identified from the 2001 infoUSA Inc. database: *57,000 Physicians and Surgeons Directory.* No independent efforts were made to validate the physician list. Another limitation of this paper was the PCP's time was not adjusted for actual time in clinic. All physicians were treated as if they were full-time at the addresses provided. No adjustments were made for physicians who are engaged full-time in research, administration or teaching, are graduates of foreign medical schools who are not citizens or lawful permanent U.S. residents, who practice exclusively in inpatient care, or whose Medicare or Medicaid licenses have been suspended for a period of 18 months or more. In addition, no adjustments were made for interns and residents, semi-retired physicians who operate a reduced practice, or graduates of foreign medical schools who do not have unrestricted licenses to practice medicine. While these limitations are problematic, overall, each would have the effect of understating the actual population-to-physician ratio.

Conclusions. Restructuring of the state/county responsibilities for HPSA designation is long overdue. Use of GIS as a required methodology would help ensure that all areas in any state that meet the intent of federal legislation and criteria of health professions shortage areas are eligible for federal consideration and designation. While these analyses reflect the robustness of GIS as a methodology for identifying geographic area HPSAs according to federal criteria, additional fine-tuning is needed to validate the results. The proposed policy change would result in more accurate information, target additional federal resources to those areas that are in greatest need, provide comprehensive data that would allow for analysis of its effectiveness, and be a more effective tool in efforts to attain 100% access and zero disparities.

REFERENCES

American Academy of Pediatrics (May 1981). Critique of the Final Report of the Graduate Medical Education National Advisory Report* (REX017. *Pediatrics* 67(5): 585-96.

Blendon, R.J., L.H. Aiken, H.E. Freeman, & C.R. Corey (1989). Access to medical care for black and white Americans: A matter of continuing concern. *Journal of the American Medical Association* 261: 278-81.

Code of Federal Regulations, Title 42, Volume 1, Parts 1 to 399, 42 CFR Part 5, 1980 (Revised as of October 1, 2000). US Government Printing Office via GPO Access.

Cornelius, L.J. (1983). Barriers to medical care for white, black, and Hispanic American children. *Journal of the National Medical Association* 85(4): 281-88.

Cornelius, L.J. (1993). Ethnic minorities and access to medical care: Where do they stand? *Journal of the Association for Academic Minority Physicians* 4(1): 16-24

Council on Graduate Medical Education. (1992). *Third Report: Improving Access to Health Care Through Physician Workforce Reform: Directions for the 21st Century.* Rockville, MD: DHHS.

Council on Graduate Medical Education (1996). *Eighth Report–Patient Care Physician Supply and Requirements: Testing COGME Recommendations.* Rockville, MD: DHHS.

Council on Graduate Medical Education (1998). *Tenth Report: Physician Distribution and Health Care Challenges in Rural and Inner-City Areas.* Washington DC: GPO.

Federal Register, Vol. 65, no. 180, September 15, 2000.

InfoUSA, Inc. (2001). *57,000 Physicians and Surgeons Directory.* Omaha, NE: infoUSA, Inc.

Lee, R.I., & Jones, L.W. (1933). *The Fundamentals of Good Medical Care–Publication of the Committee on the Costs of Medical Care,* No. 22. Chicago, IL: U. of Chicago Press.

McNutt, D.R. (1981). GMENAC its manpower forecasting framework *AJPH* 71: 1116-24.

Miller, J.I. (1967). *Report to the President of the U.S. by the National Advisory Commission on Health Manpower.* WA DC: USGPO.

Office of the President (July 1999). *Changing Directions in Medical Education. Sixth Report: 1999 Update on Systemwide Efforts to Increase the Training of Generalists.* Oakland: University of California.

Report of the National Advisory Commission on Health Manpower (1967). WA DC: USGPO.

Sec. 215 of the Public Health Service Act, 58 Stat. 690 (42 U.S.C. 216); sec. 332 of the Public Health Service Act, 90 Stat. 2270-2272 (42 U.S.C. 254e).

Smeloff, E.A., W.H. Burnett, & P.J. Kelzer (1981). A geographic framework for coordination of needs assessment for primary medical care in California. *Public Health Rep* 96: 310-4.

U.S. Department of Commerce, Bureau of Census (1990). *Census Summary File 3* (STF3A).

U.S. DHHS (1981). *Summary Report of the Graduate Medical Education National Advisory Committee*, Vol. 1, DHS Pub. No. (HRA) 18-651. WA DC: USGPO.

U.S. General Accounting Office (1978). Report to the Congress of the United States by the Comptroller General. *Are Enough Physicians of the Right Types Trained in the United States*. HRD-77-92. WA DC: USGPO.

U.S. General Accounting Office (1978). Report to the Congress of the United States by the Comptroller General. *Progress and Problems in Improving the Availability of Primary Care Providers in Underserved Areas* (HRD-77-135) WA DC: USGPO.

USDHEW (1976). *Health Manpower Issues* (HRA 76-40) WA DC: USGPO.

Wieczorek (1998). *Using Geographic Information Systems for Small Area Analysis.* Unpublished Paper.

A Study of the Influence
of Protective Factors as a Resource
to African American Males
in Traditional Batterers' Interventions

Norma Gray Jones, DSW, MSC, USN

SUMMARY. The purpose of this study was to examine the relationship between protective factors and the responses of African American males in traditional batterers' interventions. African American male batterers have been viewed as responding poorly to batterers' interventions and were reported in the literature as at risk for dropout and treatment failure. This research proposed that there were culturally related protective factors that enhanced traditional interventions for African American males, increasing their potential for changing abusive behaviors.

This within-group study used secondary data to examine the influence of protective factors on the responses of 268 active duty Navy African American males. They were a sub-sample of 861 males randomly assigned to one of four different interventions for batterers. The interventions included a cognitive behavioral men's group, couple's group, safety and stabilization group, and a control group. Each of their cases had been officially substantiated by the Navy for assault of their spouses.

Norma Gray Jones is Deputy, Fleet and Family Support Programs, Naval Personnel Command, Millington, TN.

[Haworth co-indexing entry note]: "A Study of the Influence of Protective Factors as a Resource to African American Males in Traditional Batterers' Interventions." Jones, Norma Gray. Co-published simultaneously in *Journal of Health & Social Policy* (The Haworth Press, Inc.) Vol. 16, No. 1/2, 2002, pp. 169-183; and: *Disability and the Black Community* (ed: Sheila D. Miller) The Haworth Press, Inc., 2002, pp. 169-183. Single or multiple copies of this article are available for a fee from The Haworth Document Delivery Service [1-800-HAWORTH, 9:00 a.m. - 5:00 p.m. (EST). E-mail address: docdelivery@haworthpress.com].

The measures for the protective factors of religion, self-esteem, and family support were drawn from the original study's self-report measurement tool. The results of the statistical analyses were found to be significant. The protective factors performed as social controls for reducing certain types of abusive behaviors.

Little research has been conducted on the influence of cultural factors on batterers intervention outcome for African Americans. This study established a strong support for further research. *[Article copies available for a fee from The Haworth Document Delivery Service: 1-800-HAWORTH. E-mail address: <docdelivery@haworthpress.com> Website: <http://www.HaworthPress.com> © 2002 by The Haworth Press, Inc. All rights reserved.]*

KEYWORDS. Batterers intervention, African American males, military treatment, domestic violence interventions

INTRODUCTION

The general impression is that African Americans have a low rate of participation and success in traditional batterers' treatment programs and interventions. The primary purpose of this study was to examine if there is a relationship between protective factors and the responses of African American males in traditional batterers' interventions.

Findings regarding spouse abuse in the African American community are often the results of information generated from studies where primary research questions do not address the relationships between race, culture, and responses to interventions. Considering the low level of attention given to spouse abuse in the African American community as well as to culture-based treatment and research design, this study offered an opportunity to examine culture-based characteristics of African American males and the influence upon their responses while experiencing traditional batterers' interventions (Uzzell, 1989; U.S. Dept. of Health and Human Services, 1995).

THE STUDY SAMPLE

The sample for this study originated from a randomized, longitudinal batterers' intervention study, The San Diego Navy Experiment (Dunford, 1998). The San Diego Navy Experiment was conducted with a population of active duty Navy male perpetrators of spouse abuse over a period of 18 months. There were 311 African American males representing 35% of the original study sample (N = 861). Of the 311 African American males in the study, 268 screened eligible and were selected for this within-group study sample. Over 50% of the males were between 20 and 30 years of age. Twenty-eight percent had two years or more of college, with an average monthly income of $1,871.13. The average total length of time the couples had been together was four years and three months. Fifty-five percent of the spouses reported that they worked and only 8.2 % were also on active military duty. Nearly half of the respondents had children from a prior relationship and over half had children in their current relationship as shown in Tables 1 and 2.

TABLE 1. Means, Standard Deviations, Mode and Percentages of Demographic Characteristics

N = 268	M	SD	Mode	%
Age	27.02	5.30		
Currently Married	.97			97%
Education	12.47	.98	12	
Rank	4.56		4	
Time in the Military	87.32	54.89		
Monthly Income	1871.13	574.24		
Total Monthly Income	1913.85	637.24		
Total Household Income	2526.25	1071.13		
Length of Time Married	40.59 mos. (3.4 yrs.)	35.10		
Total Time Together	50.10 mos. (4.3 yrs.)	42.42		

TABLE 2. Percentages of Spouse Employment Status and Additional Financial Resources

N = 268	Percentage	Frequency
Spouses' Employment	55.2%	148
Spouses' Active Duty Status	8.2%	22
Welfare Recipient	11.6%	31

AFRICAN AMERICAN MALES AND DOMESTIC VIOLENCE

African American males, along with the majority of male batterers through-out the United States, are currently referred to batterers' interventions that follow a cognitive behavioral model (Williams, 1993). Even though the literature indicates that the success rate is low for African Americans in traditional treatment programs, traditional batterers' interventions continue to be the most utilized resource for this population (Jones, 2001). The assumption is that all batterers can be referred to the same types of treatment programs, ignoring the relevance of culture (Williams, 1994). Examining protective factors as a resource for African American male batterers in traditional batterers' interventions provides an important step in addressing the gap in social work practice and theory and appropriately meeting the needs of African American male batterers.

The absence of culturally competent research designs and treatment programs for spouse abuse is a major issue in the mental health field (Hampton, 1991). Reports of African American males' participation in traditional batterers' programs indicate that there are gaps in assessments and interventions. Inclusion of culturally sensitive and competent facilitators, as well as culturally specific groups, would enhance the overall assessment and group process within the entire experience of African American males (Williams, 1993). Studies are not usually designed to examine specific factors such as the impact of years of oppression and racism upon African American males involved in incidents of spouse abuse, which are critical to a complete assessment and intervention plan (Caliber Associates, 1994; Staples, 1994). This color-blind approach is a common criticism of research on African Americans because of inaccurate information and inappropriate responses (Jones, 2001).

Examining African American batterers' success would encourage examination of the interventions more closely. For example, which African American males complete traditional batterers' interventions? What personal and character resources appear to be related to successful outcomes? Is there a relationship between self-esteem and response to interventions? Is there a relationship between religious beliefs and response to interventions? Is there a relationship between family support and response to interventions?

PROTECTIVE FACTORS

Family violence among African Americans must be examined in the context of strength factors (Hampton, 1994). African Americans are a diverse population who have developed a survival system based on individual, family, and community strengths. They include but are not limited to employment and education, extended family support, spiritual and religious relationships, and self-esteem (Boyd-Franklin, 1990; Staples, 1994). Sub-cultural values and beliefs can serve as barriers to seeking help or as supports and strengths. The African American families' survival and problem-solving system includes factors that, if not fully understood, could greatly impact the helping process. The absence of these factors or stress in these areas may contribute to spouse abuse (Tolman, 1990). The literature supports the idea that these factors decrease the probability of violence in families (Stith, 1990).

Family violence research has identified various internal and external factors as having a relationship between an increase and decrease in incidents of spouse abuse. They have been categorized as risk factors or protective factors for spouse abuse. For example, unemployment and poverty have been identified as risk factors of spouse abuse, and employment and family support have been identified as protective factors of spouse abuse (Straus, 1995). This study addressed protective factors and their influence as a resource for African American males in traditional batterers' interventions.

Protective factors "reflect positive mechanisms or processes that reduce the effects of negative processes associated with risk factors. They buffer the effects of risk factors on outcomes such that "relations between risks and outcomes are weaker for those with protective factors" (Voydanoff, 1999). Protective factors are resources that can be categorized into several areas: financial or economic, education and cognitive abilities, health, and character or personality resources (Stith, 1990; McCubbin, 1983).

Examining the primary strengths that serve as protective factors for African Americans can provide a conceptual framework for social work practice that includes cultural components. This approach provides an Afrocentric perspective to a program level of responses for individuals, families, and communities addressing family violence, and African American males and families.

The literature endorses family support, religion, and self-esteem as protective factors that have the potential to influence the responses that African American males experience to traditional batterers' interventions. When these factors register as high or strong, they have the potential to serve as resources enhancing one's ability to heal.

The most significant influence on decrease in spouse violence for African American families is the presence of extended family members in the home and area (Cazenave & Straus, 1995). These findings are significant in examining protective factors that consist of strengths and resources for the African American family. Protective factors serve as buffers for violence or support for problem solving.

African American Males and Response to Interventions

African American males are portrayed throughout the literature as persons who are resistant to psychological and counseling services (Thomas, 1972; Jones, 1983). These behaviors have been labeled and a description has been established without the resources or benefits of a cultural perspective. The reality of the impact of a history filled with hostility and racism has contributed to African American males becoming private and non-trusting of clinical and research settings (Jones, 1983; Davis, 1989; Akbar, 1991a). In order to respond positively to help, one's belief system must be taken into consideration (Aponte, 2000).

It has only been within recent years that an examination of the appropriateness of culture specific methods and techniques has been considered. African Americans were described as geographically unique, not culturally unique, such as in this assessment: "the peculiarities in the disease of Negroes are so distinctive that they can be safely and successfully treated . . . only by Southern physicians" (Thomas, 1972).

Culture is critical in the assessments, evaluations, and interventions formulated in the problem-solving process for African Americans and bears greatly upon intervention outcomes (Pinderhuges, 1998). This includes the awareness of racism and its influence upon life stressors. Personal problems do not negate the presence and impact of racial and gender discrimination.

The coping mechanisms developed by African American males to confront the racism and barriers encountered have hindered the development of a self-confident, assertive, and empowered masculine role. These coping mechanisms may present as an issue in intimate relationships as well as in counseling settings.

THEORETICAL FRAMEWORK

There is no one theoretical framework that currently explains the responses of African American males in traditional batterers' interventions, just as there is no one theory that explains the causes of family violence among any population (Gelles, 1980; Straus, 1979). In this study, traditional theories were examined from an Afrocentric paradigm. The study provided a culturally sensitive perspective with which to explore the behaviors of African American males.

Social Control Theory was selected because it was a concept that suggested a balance between conflict and compromise. This study took the position of using social control to examine controls for conformity. Social Control Theory provides a strengths-based perspective with which to examine the responses to interventions of African American batterers that includes a comprehensive culturally sensitive assessment, intervention, and prevention approach. This perspective offers possible explanations of the influence of African American families upon interrupting the cycle of family violence in the African American community. Functions of both choice and social exchange theories operate within Social Control Theory.

Choice and social exchange concepts are active concepts in control theory. Choice and social exchange theories deal with concepts of dependency, benefits, and choices, as well as cost and rewards. This position is supported by the studies examined in Nye's work of marital and couple relationships and the exchanges that occur to maintain continuous interactions (Nye, 1978; Nye, 1980; Davis, 1993). In African American families, there are certain factors that have been identified as significant to their sense of self, identity, success, and survival in an environment that has consciously produced hostility and interruptions (Chestang, 1980; Hampton, 1991). These protective factors represent cultural strengths and stability. Religion, family support, and self-esteem are the protective factors central to this study. They represent social control variables influencing how African Americans relate to others. Based on the strengths of the African American family, maintaining an affectionate and supportive relationship is valuable and reinforces the need to maintain an attachment to these elements that come from within the cultural system.

PROTECTIVE FACTORS AS SOCIAL CONTROLS

Characteristics of the strong and organized African American family are strong kinship bonds, commitment to work and education, and commitment to religious and spiritual participation (Lum, 1999; Aponte, 1994; Boyd-Franklin, 1990). This organized family system provides cultural resources to its members that reinforce a strong self-concept through a sense of belonging and connectedness, self-sufficiency, and positive identity as an African American (Aponte, 2000; Jackson, 1980). Positive self-concept acts as an internal source of control and promotes positive behaviors that work towards maintaining close attachments.

This study has suggested that protective factors serve as a form of social control, increasing African American males' potential for success in traditional batterers' interventions. The protective factors of religion, family support, and self-esteem are resources that have provided internal and external management of African American lives during some of the most difficult periods (Stith, 1990; McCubbin, 1983). The protective factors of family support, religion, and self-esteem were examined as elements of direct forms of social control. They function as indirect, internalized, and alternative forms of social controls. As mentioned earlier, they overlap functionally between the various forms of social control.

INSTRUMENTS

This secondary data analysis addressed the question: Do African American males who have strong protective factors have a positive response in traditional batterers' interventions?

The hypotheses for this study were formed on the relationship between the protective factors, self-esteem, religion and family support, and the responses of African American males in traditional batterers' interventions as indicated by dependent variables that were measures of abusive behavior.

The survey instrument was developed to measure the protective factors, religion, family support, and self-esteem. It consisted of 20 items drawn from the 313-item San Diego Domestic Study Questionnaire. The independent variables were selected based on the literature support of the influence of these variables on survival and problem solving for African Americans (McCubbin & Figley, 1983; McCubbin et al., 1998; Stith, Williams & Rosen, 1990; Voydanoff & Donnelly, 1999). The dependent variables were selected from the outcome measures from the San Diego Navy Experiment. Nine factors or sub-scales were developed from the 42 items of the Conflict Tactic Scale (CTS) and identified as the Modified Conflict Tactic Scale (MCTS), which measures the presence and types of abusive behaviors (Dunford, 1998). The outcome measures used were the female victim's response to the MCTS. They were interviewed individually, as were each of the male participants. The nine outcome measures were broken down between episodic measures, which indicated frequency of abuse, and MCTS, which focused on the different types of abusive behaviors that occurred. The literature suggests that it is the victim's report of abusive behavior that is the most accurate (Straus, 1979). High scores indicate high levels of abuse. Interventions were conducted for a total of 12 months. The outcome measures from the second and third waves (conducted every 6 months) were combined to reflect this period of data analyzed. This study was designed to test for the existence of a negative relationship between protective factors and battering behaviors of African American males in traditional batterers' interventions.

RESULTS

The relationship between the protective factors and the outcome variables were examined utilizing Pearson Correlation coefficients. Correlations between nine continuous and three dichotomous predictors were conducted. There were 18 statistically significant correlations found at the 0.05 level (one-tailed) out of a possible 108 (Table not shown). The strength of the correlation coefficient was small for all identified correlations, however, statistical significance was found. The significant relationships found between total time lived together and time lived together in the last six months, and the outcome variables, suggest that these two independent variables serve as protective factors for African American males during the traditional batterers' interventions. There is a pattern of activity and support for a relationship between the protective factors and a decrease in certain abusive behaviors as suggested by the hypotheses. The greatest Pearson's correlation coefficients calculated in this set of correlations was for Total time together and Misdemeanor abuse, r $(-219) = -.2$, which was negative and statistically significant. Statistical significance was found at the .05 (one-tailed) level, the strength of the correlation was small. For that reason and in the presence of the other variables, linear regression analysis was conducted to determine if the variables continue to come up in the presence of other variables. The second step utilized linear regression analyses to examine how much abuse occurred (Table 3).

Several predictors under the family support variable were combined to reduce redundancy. The following variables were collapsed: Family too far away to help was collapsed into How stressful not having family close; Separated in the last six months was collapsed into How stressful separation; Cur-

TABLE 3. Linear Regression Analyses of Protective Factors and Outcome Measures

N = 218	Felony Abuse			Misdemeanor Abuse		
	B	∃	t	B	∃	t
Attend Church?	−0.009	−.019	−.262	−7.900	−.061	−.850
Important Religion?	−0.032	−.068	−.945	−3.892	−.031	−.435
His Self-esteem?	−0.008	−.063	−.893	−3.672	−.106	−1.517
Stress family not close?	−0.049	−.128	−1.859	−9.377	−.095	−1.380
Stress separation?	0.018	.052	.680	3.817	.042	.563
# together 6 months?	0.007	.024	.324	−4.608	−.057	−.760
Total # together?	−0.003	−.190	−2.781*	−8.178	−.224	−3.315*
# talked about problem?	0.004	.127	1.817	2.655	.035	.506
	R = .079*, F = (2.199)*			R^2 = .078*, F = (2.228)*		

*Significant, p < .05
Dependent variables are log-transformed

rently married and How long married were collapsed into Amount of time living together in the last six months. Based on the literature, these were theoretically the best measures for the family support variables from the data available. The linear regression revealed less activity than the correlation analyses. Two models out of a possible nine showed statistical significance, misdemeanor ($R^2 = .078$), and felony abuse ($R^2 = .079$). Only 8% of the variance in misdemeanor abuses could be explained by the combined protective factors, and only 8% of the variances in felony abuses could be explained by the combined protective factors. The statistical significance found in the linear regression models, though small, supports some of the relationships identified in the correlation analyses. There was negative and statistical significance found in the family support factors. These findings suggest that the protective factor of family support, and specifically total time together, have an influence on abusive behaviors. The more time the couple had been together, the less felony and misdemeanor abuses were found.

Examining the actual chance of abuse occurring was the next analysis conducted (see Table 4). The logistic regression analysis was conducted to identify the probability of abuse occurring based on the relationship between the independent and dependent variables. There was statistical significance found in the models for fear, injury, felony, menacing, and passive abuses. There was statistical significance in five models out of a possible nine. Total time together and self-esteem were most frequently identified as statistically significant in whether or not abuse would occur. The analyses suggest that these two variables serve as protective factors, and that less abuse would occur with increased self-esteem and length of relationship. The more time together that a couple has, the less likely certain types of abusive behaviors will occur. The higher the self-esteem, the less likely certain types of abusive behaviors will occur.

These findings directly support Hypothesis 1 and Hypothesis 3. Self-esteem and family support serve as protective factors for African American males in traditional batterers' interventions, reducing certain types of abusive behaviors.

The results of this study did support Hypothesis 1: The higher the self-esteem of African American males, the greater the reduction in abusive behaviors while in traditional batterers' interventions; and Hypothesis 3: The stronger the family support, the greater the reduction in abusive behaviors while in traditional batterers' interventions.

This study did not support Hypothesis 2: The stronger the religious attachment or belief of African American males, the greater the reduction in abusive behaviors while in traditional batterers' interventions.

TABLE 4. Logistic Regression Models, Frequency of Abuse Reported by Female Victims

N = 218	FR B	IJ B	FEL B	MIS B	PAS B
Attend Church?	−.0444	−.2472	.0531	−.2292	−.3558
Important Religion?	−.0993	−.0859	.2322	.0819	−.2734
Stress family not close?	−.1124	−.0889	.0882	−.0077	−.2927*
Stress separation?	.1393	.0503	.0352	.0201	−.2379
# talked about problem?	.0008	.0085	.0075	−.0009	.1567
# together 6 months?	−.0755	−.1245	.0115	−.1020	−.1941
Total # together?	−.0047	−.0152*	.0203*	−.0089*	−.0114*
# Self-esteem?	−.0890*	−.0105	.0520	−.0951*	−.0407
R^2	.054*	.069*	.06*	.09*	.14*

*Significant, $p < .05$

DISCUSSION

This study, the first of its kind, was selected out of ethical concerns and application needs to address the consistent reports of African American males' poor responses and failures in traditional batterers' interventions (Williams, 1995b). This is a problem that not only exists in the civilian community but also in the United States Navy. Nye's Social Control Theory was used to examine three factors that have historically served as sources of strength and motivation for African Americans: religion, self-esteem, and family support; two of three hypotheses tested were found to be significant. *The higher the self-esteem of African American males, the greater the reduction in abusive behaviors.* This research supports Nye and Gelles' theoretical position that high self-esteem can be interpreted as indicative of the respondents feeling good about themselves, including their ethnic and racial backgrounds. Further, the finding of high self-esteem suggests the respondents' investment in self as well as an internal need to maintain certain attachments and relationships of value, thus influencing behavior to support this (Nye, 1980; Gelles, 1981). Aponte (2000) has noted that high self-esteem allows one to call upon internal resources when needed, again supporting the influence of high self-esteem as a social control. Thus, self-esteem serves to regulate the respondents' behavior, as in the reduction of abuse (Gelles, 1981). Under these circumstances, these protective factors function as social controls.

The second hypothesis, *The stronger the religious beliefs of African American males, the greater the reduction in abusive behaviors,* was not found to be significant. The literature suggests a strong and influential relationship between religion and the lives of African Americans in general. However, there was no literature support specific to the role and influence of religion on abusive behaviors of African American males (Staples, 1993; Hill, 1997; Gary et al., 1984). It may be that the measurements in this study were not sensitive enough to address this issue.

The third hypothesis, *The stronger the family supports for African American males, the greater the reduction in abusive behaviors*, was supported. There were five measures analyzed for family support. This study found that the length of the couple's relationship functions as an element of social control. It can be argued that the longer the couple's relationship, the greater the potential for the relationship to function as a protective factor. These findings suggest that the longer the relationship, the greater the investment to maintain the relationship. According to Nye's Social Control Theory, the investment in the relationship becomes an indirect element of social control. The risk of losing the relationship becomes the motivation for changing behaviors that may place the relationship in jeopardy, such as abuse (Nye, 1980). The various constructs used in this study to measure this aspect of family support demonstrated a reduction in fear, hitting, menacing, felony, controlling, passive, and misdemeanor abuses the longer the couple had been together.

This study supports already existing theoretical and empirical evidence for a relationship between family and friends acting as an element of social control, resulting in a decrease in family violence (Nye, 1979).

The study has taken steps to engage research in an area that has been avoided. There have been numerous studies conducted on interventions for batterers and typologies of batterers. These two areas have failed to examine African Americans separately from large mixed populations. The unique and individual personality characteristics and psychological makeup of African Americans demand that they be studied in a manner that includes their perspectives and their culture. To continue to ignore this need is to avoid taking responsibility for their continued poor response to traditional interventions. This study has demonstrated that there are cultural factors that intervene in how African Americans specifically respond to traditional interventions for batterers. In future studies that are conducted, it is the ethical responsibility for those who have established themselves as the experts in this field to take responsibility for inclusion of African Americans within the unique characteristics of their culture.

This study argues against current accepted practice standards for batterers' interventions for African American males. It has demonstrated the wisdom for inclusion of cultural factors, which would elicit valid and reliable responses from batterers from different backgrounds. These findings suggest an option to the "one size fits all" approach for responding to batterers. These options place emphasis on the social work value of starting "where the client is." The findings from this study further suggest the importance of utilizing the person-in-the-environment perspective. It requires responding to the needs of the batterer as opposed to making the batterer fit into a prepackaged response.

As noted earlier, this research is a secondary data analysis, which presents with obvious the limitations of using data not specifically designed for the study in focus.

This study raises the issue of the significance of protective factors as a focus for batterers' interventions regardless of family origin and culture. The statistical activity generated in this study included trends that strongly suggest the assumptions that generated the hypotheses are well worth further exploration.

REFERENCES

Akbar, N. (1991a). The evolution of human psychology for African Americans. In R. L. Jones (Ed.), *Black Psychology* (3rd ed., pp. 99-124). Berkeley, CA: Cobb and Henry Publishers.

Aponte, H. (1994). *Bread and Spirit: Therapy with the New Poor.* New York, NY: Morton Press.

Aponte, H. (2000). Influence of one's culture on their response to interventions: unpublished.

Boyd-Franklin, N. (1990). Five key factors in the treatment of black families. In K. V. Hardy (Ed.), *Minorities and Family Therapy.* New York, NY: The Haworth Press, Inc.

Caliber Associates (1994). *Preliminary Process Study Report* (CDRL No. A003 D.O. 5005 of Contract No. F49650-92-D5006). Washington, DC: Department of Defense.

Cazenave, N. A., & Straus, M. A. (1995). Race, class, network embeddedness and family violence: A Search for potent support systems. In M. A. Straus & R. J. Gelles (Eds.), *Physical Violence in American Families: Risk Factors and Adaptations to Violence in 8,145 Families* (pp. 321). New Brunswick, NJ: Transaction Publishers.

Chestang, L. (1980). Character development in a hostile environment. In M. Bloom (Ed.), *Life Span Development: Bases for Preventive and Interventive Helping (pp. 40-50).* New York, NY: Macmillan Publishers.

Davis, L. E. (1993). *Black and Single.* Chicago, IL: Noble Press.

Davis, L. E., & Proctor, E. K. (1989). *Race, Gender and Class.* Englewood Cliffs, NJ: Prentice Hall.

Dunford, F. W. (1998). *The San Diego Navy Experiment: An Experimental Assessment of Interventions for Men Who Assault Their Wives.* Boulder, CO: University of Colorado.

Dunford, F. W. (2000). The San Diego Navy experiment: An assessment of interventions for men who assault their wives. *Journal of Consulting and Clinical Psychology, 68*(3), 468-476.

Gary, L. E. (1991). Mental health of African Americans: Research trends and directions. In R. L. Jones (Ed.), *Black Psychology* (3rd ed.). Berkeley, CA: Cobb and Henry Publishers.

Gelles, R. J. (1980). Violence in the family: A review of research in the seventies. *Journal of Marriage and the Family*, *42*, 873-86.

Gelles, R. J. (1981). An exchange social control theory. In D. Finkelhor, R. J. Gelles, G. T. Hotaling, & M. A. Straus (Eds.), *The Dark Side of Families (pp.151-165)*. Thousand Oaks, CA: Sage Publications.

Gelles, R. J., & Straus, M. A. (1979). Determinants of violence in the family: Towards a theoretical integration. In W. R. Burr, R. Hill, F. I. Nye, & I. L. Reiss (Eds.), *Contemporary Theories About the Family (pp. 549-581)*. New York, NY: The Free Press.

Hampton, R. G., Gelles, R. J., & Harrop, J. W. (1989). Is violence in black families increasing? A comparison of 1975 and 1985 national survey rates. *Journal of Marriage and the Family*, *51*, 969-980.

Hampton, R. L. (1991). *Black Family Violence: Current Research and Theory*. Lexington, KY: Lexington Books.

Hampton, R. L., & Gelles, R. J. (1994). Violence toward black women in a nationally representative sample of Black American families. *Journal of Comparative Family Studies*, *25*, 105-120.

Hill, R. B. (1997). *The Strengths of African American Families: Twenty-Five Years Later* (2nd ed.). Washington, DC: R&B Publisher.

Jackson, J. S., Tucker, M. B., & Gurin, G. (1980). *National Survey of Black Americans (Machine Readable data file)*. Ann Arbor, MI: Institute for Social Research, Distributor: Inter-University Consortium for Political and Social Research.

Jones, B., & Gay, B. (1983). Black males and psychotherapy. *American Journal of Psychotherapy*, *37*, 77-85.

Jones, N. G. (May 2001). A study of the influence of protective factors on the response of african american males in traditional batterers interventions. In *A Population of Active Duty Male Batterers*, Accepted for Publication (Doctoral Dissertation, Norfolk State University 2001).

Lum, D. (1999). *Social Work Practice and People of Color: A process stage approach*. Canada: Wadsworth.

McCubbin, H., & Figley, C. (1983). *Stress and the Family: Coping with Normative Transitions*. (Vol. 1). New York, NY: Bruner and Mazel.

McCubbin, H. I., Thompson, E. A., Thompson, A. I., & Futrell, J. A. (Eds.) (1998). *Resiliency in African American Families*. Thousand Oaks, CA: Sage Publications.

Nobles, W. (1991). African philosophy: Foundations for black psychology. In R. Jones (Ed.), *Black Psychology* (3rd ed.) (pp.47-64). Berkeley, CA: Cobb and Henry Publishers.

Nye, F. I. (1978). Is choice and exchange theory the key? *Journal of Marriage and the Family*, *40*(2), 219-233.

Nye, F. I. (1980). Family mini theories as special instances of choice and exchange theory. *Journal of Marriage and the Family*, *42*(3), 479-489.

Pinderhuges, E. (1998). Black genealogy revisited. In M. McGoldrick (Ed.), *Re-Visioning Family Therapy*. New York, NY: The Guilford Press.

Staples, R. (1994). *Black Families: Essays and Studies* (5th ed.). New York, NY: Van Nostrand Reinhold.

Stith, S., Williams, M., & Rosen, K. (Eds.) (1990). *Violence Hits Home: Comprehensive Treatment Approaches to Domestic Violence*. New York, NY: Springer.

Straus, M. A. (1979). Measuring intrafamily conflict and violence. *Journal of Marriage and the Family, 41*, 75-88.

Straus, M. A. (1990). The conflict tactic scales and its critics: an evaluation and new data on validity and reliability. In R. A. Gelles & M. A. Straus (Eds.), *Physical Violence in American Families*, 49-73. New Brunswick, NJ: Transactions Publisher.

Straus, M. A., & Gelles, R. J. (1986). Societal change and change in family violence from 1975 to 1985 as revealed by two national surveys. *Journal of Marriage and the Family, 48*, 465-479.

Thomas, A., & Sillen, S. (1972). *Racism and Psychiatry* (Carol Publishing Group, 1993, ed.). Secaucus, NJ: Carol Publishing Group.

Tolman, R. M., & Edleson, J. L. (1995). Intervention for men who batter, A review of research. In S. M. Stith & M. A. Straus (Eds.), *Understanding Partner Violence* (pp. 262-270). Minneapolis, MN: National Council on Family Relations.

Tolman, R. T., & Bennett, L. (1990). A review of quantitative research on men who batter. *Journal of Interpersonal Violence, 5*(1), 87-118.

U.S. Dept. of Health and Human Services (1995, May 31-June 2, 1995). *Institute on Domestic Violence in the African American Community*. Paper presented at the Institute on Domestic Violence in the African American Community, Minneapolis, MN.

Uzzell, O., & Peebles-Wilkins, W. (1989). Black spouse abuse: A focus on relational factors and intervention strategies. *The Western Journal of Black Studies, 13*(1), 12-15.

Voydanoff, P., & Donnelly, B. W. (1999). Risk and protective factors for psychological adjustment and grades among adolescents. *Journal of Family Issues, 20*(3), 328-349.

Williams, O. (1995). Working in groups with african american men who batter. In L. Davis (Ed.), *Working with African American Males* (pp. 229-242). Thousand Oaks, CA: Sage Publications.

Williams, O. J. (1993). Developing an African American perspective to reduce spouse abuse: Considerations for community action. *Black Caucus: Journal of the National Association of Black Social Workers, 1*(2), 1-8.

Williams, O. J., & Becker, L. R. (1994). Domestic violence partner abuse treatment programs and cultural competence: The results of a national survey. *Violence and Victims, 9*(3), 287-296.

African Centered Family Healing:
An Alternative Paradigm

Elijah Mickel, DSW, CRT, LICSW

SUMMARY. African centered family healing posits an alternative paradigm that can be used as a model for family healing. Effective intervention begins with the recognition that what we have been doing has not been working for African American families (Boyd-Franklin, 1989; Kambon, 1998; Logan, Freeman and McRoy, 1990; Owusu-Bempah, 1999; and Weaver, 1992). Social work intervention efforts must integrate mental health constructs that exist in the communities we are attempting to serve. One such concept is communal knowledge. Another such concept is communal values. When one joins communal knowledge and values, one begins to restructure the understanding of mental health in the African American family. The family unit must be viewed as interdependent. This understanding is requisite to family healing. It is therefore necessary that we change our thinking and then our actions. This article posits that social workers must become social healers. *[Article copies available for a fee from The Haworth Document Delivery Service: 1-800-HAWORTH. E-mail address: <docdelivery@haworthpress.com> Website: <http://www.HaworthPress.com> © 2002 by The Haworth Press, Inc. All rights reserved.]*

KEYWORDS. African centered, disability, family, fun, gender, harmony, healing, interdependence, Kuumba, Maat, polarity, reciprocity, social healers, teachability

---

Elijah Mickel is Professor, Delaware State University.

[Haworth co-indexing entry note]: "African Centered Family Healing: An Alternative Paradigm." Mickel, Elijah. Co-published simultaneously in *Journal of Health & Social Policy* (The Haworth Press, Inc.) Vol. 16, No. 1/2, 2002, pp. 185-193; and: *Disability and the Black Community* (ed: Sheila D. Miller) The Haworth Press, Inc., 2002, pp. 185-193. Single or multiple copies of this article are available for a fee from The Haworth Document Delivery Service [1-800-HAWORTH, 9:00 a.m. - 5:00 p.m. (EST). E-mail address: docdelivery@haworthpress.com].

http://www.haworthpress.com/store/product.asp?sku=J045
10.1300/J045v16n01_15

The clue to community can be found in the inner creative activity of living substances.

–Howard Thurman

INTRODUCTION

This article presents an African centered paradigm. This article is constructed to address mental health rather than illness, which provides a framework that contributes to the understanding of the African centered approach to family mental health (Kambon, 1998). Mental disorders have "substantial" cost for individuals, families and communities (Kessler, Abelson and Zhao, 1998). Family is the operative level of intervention because whether one works with individuals, communities, groups or organizations, intervention is always with the family. A significant focus for disability treatment in families is in the area of mental disorders. According to NIMH (2001), "Mental disorders are common in the United States and internationally. An estimated 22.1 percent of Americans ages 18 and older–about 1 in 5 adults–suffer from a diagnosable mental disorder in a given year. When applied to the 1998 U.S. Census residential population estimate, this figure translates to 44.3 million people. In addition, 4 of the 10 leading causes of disability in the U.S. and other developed countries are mental disorders . . . "

This model uses an African centered foundation for understanding human behavior. It presents a model that can be used by social workers and other healers to integrate practice skills with family strengths (Hill, 1972, 1997), through the use of the Black perspective. In order to improve intervention, we must expand our vision of both the client and the treatment providers (Mickel, 1999). The vision of the family must focus on interdependence as central to healing. The vision of the social worker must be that of the healer (Mickel, 1997).

MENTAL DISORDERS

The healing perspective is inclusive and gives priority to all members of the national and international community who were and continue to be oppressed. The very act of sanctioning the healing perspective raises to the conscious level the perception that the struggle to end oppression is not over. According to Wilson (1993, p. 3), "In the context of a racist social system, psychological diagnosis, labeling and treatment of the behavior of politically oppressed persons are political acts performed to attain political ends. For oppression begins as a psychological fact and is in good part a psychological state. If oppression is to operate with maximum efficiency, it must become and remain a psychological condition . . . " The healing perspective provides the lens though which to view the traditional political definition of mental disorders.

The very act of defining mental disorders occurs within the oppressive environment of pathology. According to the American Psychiatric Association (1994, p. xxi), "[a]lthough this manual provides a classification of mental disorders, it must be admitted that no definition adequately specifies precise boundaries for the concept of 'mental disorder.' The concept of mental disorder, like many other concepts in medicine and science, lacks a consistent operational definition that covers all situations." This inconsistent approach to delimiting the parameters of "disorder" allows practitioners to creatively define mental disorders. Definitions precede the treatment models and methods. Traditional treatments ignore the continuing research which questions treatment effectiveness (Bickman, Summerfelt and Noser, 1997). It is necessary for the competent practitioner to use this knowledge to become a social healer of mental disorders.

SOCIAL WORKERS TO SOCIAL HEALERS

Practitioners of social healing must also be able to evaluate and apply relevant theories. Their theoretical and practice parameters play a significant role in the forming of social workers' (healers') interventions. According to Armah (1973, p. 202), "Since how many seasons gone have we needed healers to reveal to us the secret of all healers' work? The body that is whole moves always together. No part of it goes against any other part. That has never been a mystery to us." The holistic parameter provides a frame of reference within which subsequent treatment occurs. Our external acts result from internal attitudes (Karass and Glasser, 1980). This process is essential to effectively integrating specific theory with practice. Mental health as an interdependent process requires understanding connecting constructs that exist in family systems.

Many social workers have not viewed family mental health as interdependent. Family mental health has generally utilized the traditional model for understanding family (Everett, Chipungu and Leashore, 1991). Many of the traditional approaches ignore the rich heritage of diverse cultures. The traditional paradigm shift (Schriver, 1998) is merely the mixing of old methods with "new" materials to achieve "old" outcomes. It is a process similar to placing old wine in a new wineskin.

African centered family mental healing includes knowledge, values and skills that enhance the well-being of people and assist in ameliorating environmental conditions that adversely affect people. This paradigm includes theory and knowledge about the family that is significant to a holistic understanding between spiritual, social, psychological and cultural systems.

AFRICAN CENTERED HEALING PARADIGM

African centered family mental healing provides a structure that reaffirms what many practitioners would do both historically as well as intuitively. The African centered world view (Mickel, 1991, 1994, 1995, and West, 1993) approaches human behavior as an interdependent relationship between the mind, body and spirit. It is a holistic approach that recognizes and supports interdependence. The primary objective of African centered family mental healing is to liberate the individual from the limits of the constricting environment. Historically, disabilities (mental disorders) have been viewed as constricting. According to Thurman (1986, p. 5), "In the human society, the experience of community, in realized potential, is rooted in life itself because the intuitive human urge for community reflects a characteristic of all life." African centered family mental health expands the parameters within which families are able to increase perceptual choices, while at the same time maintaining harmonious relationship with their perceptual world. This is the logic of wellness.

The logic of wellness from an African centered perspective involves the union of opposites (McMahon, 1990). This logic posits that all sets are interrelated through mental, physical and spiritual networks and the highest value is in interpersonal spiritual relationships. A goal of mental health intervention is to promote reconciliation, settlement, compromise, or understanding. African centered family wellness must include reciprocity as an outcome. According to Armah (1973, p. 17), "Reciprocity. Not merely taking, not merely offering. Giving, but only to those from whom we receive in equal measure. Receiving, but only from those to whom we give in reciprocal measure."

Reciprocity is especially significant for African centered family healers. According to Karenga (1990, p. 91) "The law of reciprocity, he teaches, insures that what is done to others will be done to you; thus, he says the robber will end up being robbed and the conspirator entrapped by his/her own means." The establishment of an interdependent, interpersonal relationship requires that one seek harmony, truth as well as social and economic justice. Relationships are based on natural laws that include justice, truth and reciprocity. It is best expressed in the historic search for Maat. Karenga (1990, p. 93) states, "Maat above all is truth, justice, righteousness. Justice, then, starts at the heart of what it means to follow MAAT and create a Maatian moral community. And justice begins with respecting the human person and giving her (him) her (his) due. In African ethics, shared social wealth is essential." An ethical foundation is required in order to promote reconciliation of opposing parties.

The African centered paradigm (Mickel, 1991, 1994, 1995, 2000; Mickel and Liddie-Hamilton, 1998) explicates interdependence as the essential principle that must be correlated with the basic needs. Mental disorder healing is a change process involving a number of change systems. The first system is comprised of the consumer(s), the second system is the healer, and the third is the mental health environment where the change (healing) occurs. The consumer(s) and the healers bring their cultural and ethnic uniqueness to the mental health environment. For example, those who would work in the African American community need to recognize the dual perspective. This perspective has posited that the Africans in America are both African and "American." In this instance, the author uses the common misconception that "American" means a citizen of the United States. The truth is "American" is any citizen of two continents. As we begin to heal, truth in definitions is a requisite. Effective intervention requires the development of a need-fulfilling environment. The need-fulfilling environment provides the loci where restructuring of the intervention process occurs. There is a continuum of proximal-distal cause effect relationships. Community-based treatment by nature includes a focus on social conditions as significant causes of mental disorders. The traditional research approaches focus on looking for proximal causes. The more holistic approach focuses upon distal causes. Proximal causes exist within the distal causes. From this frame of reference, both empirical and axiological questions must be addressed. Modern epistemology and its concomitant axiology focuses attention on proximate, individually-based risk factors, and away from social conditions as causes of disease (Link and Phelan, 1995). This paradigm guides our understanding of an African worldview which is essential when working from an African centered paradigm. African centered family healing, can be explicated under each level, although this paper emphasizes the concepts of teachability, fun, kuumba, polarity and gender as explainers. (See Chart 1.)

The principle of polarity posits that all behavior exists on a continuum. This principle provides a strong rationale for intervention in the family system. If one understands the presenting problem, the solution is also near. All problems as well as solutions exist along the same continuum, therefore every problem has a solution and this solution is inherent to the problem. According to the Three Initiates (1988, p. 125), "Everything is dual; everything has poles; everything has its pair of opposites; like and unlike are the same; opposites are identical in nature, but different in degree; extremes meet; all truths are but half-truths; all paradoxes may be reconciled."

A second principle of duality is Gender which is a principle which describes creation. It occurs at all levels and is manifested through the union of oppo-

CHART 1. African Centered Healing Paradigm

PHILOSOPHY	BASIC NEEDS	NGUZO SABA	HERMETIC PRINCIPLES
ESSENTIALITY OF MORAL SOCIAL PRACTICE	LOVE	UMOJA	CORRESPONDENCE
FREEWILL	FREEDOM	KUJICHA-GULIA	CAUSE/EFFECT
PERFECTIBILITY	POWER	UJIMA/NIA/ UJAMAA	VIBRATION RHYTHM
TEACHABILITY	FUN	KUUMBA	POLARITY GENDER
DIVINE IMAGE	SPIRITUAL	IMANI	MENTALISM

sites. Each issue has two poles. According to the Three Initiates (1988, p. 148), "The office of Gender is solely that of creating, producing, generating, etc., and its manifestations are visible on every plane of phenomena."

The teachability of humans posits that people are teachable and capable of moral cultivation which leads to his or her high self. The goal of teaching is wisdom based upon morality. Morality is defined by one's family and community. Teachability recognizes the value of information and knowledge as key processes in choosing behavior (which, after all, is based upon perception).

Kuumba (creativity) is the essential component in the restoration, healing and repairing of oppressed people. Families, creatively, fashion a way of coping within a rejecting society. It is through this process that restructuring occurs. We use the African centered process to challenge misinformation and develop a new history. According to Asante (1988, p. 6), "It is our history, our mythology, our creative motif, and our ethos exemplifying our collective will. On the basis of our story, we build upon the work of our ancestors who gave signs toward our humanizing function." Interdependence is a part of our story.

The struggle for harmony includes a perceptual acceptance that life is worth living. Families struggle for liberation, victory, love for each other, vision, values and the right to make their own decisions. Fun in essence is the (re)creational aspect of our basic needs. In order to live in an environment that we perceive as need-fulfilling there must be a time and place for re-creation (fun). It is especially important that the need for fun be addressed as an essential component of the healing process. Therefore, the healing behaviors contain two components–the obvious and the unknown. These components reflect the concept of a dual perspective. The Black family lives in two worlds. It has a double consciousness (DuBois, 1989). This double consciousness influences the treatment of illness and wellness. To be well is a reconciliation of disparity and bringing life into balance with a paradigm shift.

CONCLUSION

The foundation of this perspective is the knowledge and value system that are essential for making a shift to an African centered healing paradigm. This shift is required as one should not attempt to put new wine in old wine skins. We must develop a paradigm for understanding how some of the people we work with construct reality. This paradigm is especially useful for those who would work with African American families. In developing paradigms, we must transform our perception of both the form and function of the treatment process. That transformation begins with a review of our epistemology and axiology models.

Forward-looking thinkers must establish an African American philosophy to govern what happens to families once they become embroiled within the external system. When one works with the African American family, (s)he must use a paradigm that appreciates the struggle to overcome oppression. It must further be recognized that what is good for the African American family will be good for all families. The African centered healing paradigm provides a foundation for restructuring intervention as we move to interdependence from a holistic perspective.

REFERENCES

American Psychiatric Association (1994). *Diagnostic and statistical manual of mental disorders (fourth edition)*. Washington, DC: Author

Armah, A.K. (1973). *Two thousand seasons*. Portsmouth, NH: Heinemann Educational Books.

Bickman, L, Noser, K. and Summerfelt. W.T. (1999). Long-term effects of a system of care on children and adolescents. *The Journal of Behavioral Health Services & Research, 26*(2), 185-202.

Billingsley, A. (1992). *Climbing Jacob's ladder*. New York: Touchstone Books.

Boyd-Franklin, N. (1989). *Black families in therapy*. New York: The Guilford Press.

CSWE (1973). *Black task force*. New York: Author.

DuBois, W.E.B. (1989). *The souls of Black folk*. New York: Bantam Books.

Everett, J.E, Chipungu, S.S. and Leashore, B. R. (1991). *Child welfare: An Africentric perspective*. New Brunswick: Rutgers University Press.

Glasser, W. (1986). *Control theory in the classroom*. New York: Harper and Row.
(1965). *Reality therapy*. New York: Harper and Row.
(1972). *The identity society*. New York: Harper and Row.

Hale-Benson, J.E. (1982). *Black children*. Baltimore: Johns Hopkins University Press.

Hill, R.B. (1997). *The strengths of African American families: Twenty-five years later*. Washington, DC: R&B Publishers.

Hill, R.B. (1972). *The strengths of Black families*. New York: Emerson Hall.

Institute For Reality Therapy (1987). *Policies and procedures manual*. Los Angeles, CA: Author.

Joseph, G.G., Reddy, V. and Searle-Chatterjee, M. (1990). Eurocentrism in the social sciences. *Race and class, 31*(4), 1-24.

Kambon, K.K.K. (1998). *African/Black psychology in the American context: An African centered approach*. Tallahassee, Fl: Nubian Nation.

Karenga, M. (1990). *The book of coming forth by day*. Los Angeles: University of Sankore Press.

Karrass, C.L. and Glasser, W. (1980). *Both-win management*. New York: Lippincott & Crowell, Publishers.

Kessler, R.C., Abelson, J.M. and Zhao, S. (1998). The Epidemiology of mental disorders 3-24, in Williams, J.B.W. and Ell, K. (Editors). *Advances in mental health research: Implications for practice*. Washington, DC: NASW Press

Link, B. and Phelan, J. (1995). Social conditions as fundamental causes of disease. *Journal of Health and Social Behavior, 80-94*.

Logan, S.M.L., Freeman, E.M. and McRoy, R.G. (1990). *Social work practice with Black families*. White Plains, NY: Longman.

McMahon, M.O. (1990). *The general method of social work practice*. Englewood Cliffs, NJ: Prentice-Hall.

Mickel, E. (2000). African-Centered reality therapy: Intervention and prevention, 137-162, in Logan, S.L., and Freeman, E. M. (Editors). *Health care in the Black community*. New York: The Haworth Press, Inc.

(1995). Andragogy and control theory: Theoretical foundation for family mediation. *Journal of Reality Therapy, 14*(2), 55-62.

(1994). Control theory and the African centered perspective for quality management. *Journal of Reality Therapy, 14*(1), 49-60.

(1991). Family therapy utilizing control theory: A systems perspective. *Journal of Reality Therapy, 10*(1), 26-33.

(1993). Reality therapy based planning model. *Journal of Reality Therapy, 13*(1), 32-39.

(1999). Self-Help in African American communities: A historical review, 410-419 in Compton, B.R. and Galaway, B.

(1999). *Social work processes (6th ed.)* Pacific Grove, CA.: Brooks/Cole Publishing.

and Liddie-Hamilton (1997). Addiction, choice theory and violence: A systems approach. *Journal of Reality Therapy, 17*(1), 24-28.

and Liddie-Hamilton (1998). Black Family Therapy: Spirituality, social constructivism and choice theory. *Journal of Reality Therapy, 18*(1), 29-33.

and Mickel, C. (1999). Teaching and learning without schooling: Quality classroom case study. *International Journal of Reality Therapy, 19*(1), 39-41.

National Institute of Mental Health (2001). *The numbers count*. Bethesda, MD: Author.

Owusu-Bempah, K. (1999). Confidentiality and social work practice in African cultures, 166-170 in Compton, B.R. and Galaway, B. (1999). *Social work processes (6th ed.)*. Pacific Grove, CA.: Brooks/Cole Publishing.

Schriver, J.M. (1998). *Human behavior and the social environment*. Boston: Allyn and Bacon.

Semmes, C.E. (1981). Foundations of an Afrocentric social science: Implications of curriculum-building, theory, and research in Black Studies. *Journal of Black Studies, 12*, 3-17.

Some, M.P. (1994). *Of water and the spirit*. New York: G.P. Putnam's Sons.

Three Initiates (1988). *The kybalion*. Clayton, GA: Tri-State Press.

Thurman, H. (1986). *The search for common ground*. Richmond, IN: Friends United Press.

Weaver, H.N. (1992). African-Americans and social work: An overview of the ante-bellum through progressive eras. *Journal of Multicultural Social Work*, 2(40), 91-102.

West, C. (1993). *Keeping faith*. New York: Routledge.

Wilkinson, C.B. (Editor) (1986). *Ethnic psychiatry: Cultural issues in psychiatry*. New York: Plenum Publishing Corp.

Williams, J.B. (1998). Classification and diagnostic assessment, 25-48, in Williams, J.B.W. and Ell, K. (Editors). *Advances in mental health research: Implications for practice*. Washington, DC: NASW Press

Wilson, A.N. (1993). *The falsification of Afrikan consciousness*. New York: African World InfoSystems.

A Model Program
for African American Children
in the Foster Care System

Aminifu R. Harvey, DSW, LICSW
Georgette K. Loughney, MSW, LGSW
Janaé Moore, MSW, LCSW

SUMMARY. The children who come into shelter care are usually children who have been abused and neglected. Many have experienced numerous placements. Typically, these children have had to perform adult roles, such as caring for their own siblings or parents. They have not had the opportunity to negotiate the developmental phases of childhood in a healthy manner. Few appropriate socialization behaviors have been modeled. Many of these children demonstrate a sense of mistrust, hopelessness and serious academic problems. These are factors that have the potential to lead to life disabilities.

Based on their work in the foster care system, the authors maintain that interventions at any level in the continuum of care can contribute to the healthy development of children. Effective interventions at the shelter care level may significantly reduce the foster child's potential for lifelong disabilities. This article will focus on African American males in

Aminifu R. Harvey is Associate Professor, University of Maryland, Baltimore, MD 21201-1777 (E-mail: Aharvey@ssw.umaryland.edu). Georgette K. Loughney is Former Director, Eastern Point Children's Shelter, Annapolis, MD. Janaé Moore is Clinical Training Manager, Catholic Charities, Washington, DC.

[Haworth co-indexing entry note]: "A Model Program for African American Children in the Foster Care System." Harvey, Aminifu R., Georgette K. Loughney, and Janaé Moore. Co-published simultaneously in *Journal of Health & Social Policy* (The Haworth Press, Inc.) Vol. 16, No. 1/2, 2002, pp. 195-206; and: *Disability and the Black Community* (ed: Sheila D. Miller) The Haworth Press, Inc., 2002, pp. 195-206. Single or multiple copies of this article are available for a fee from The Haworth Document Delivery Service [1-800-HAWORTH, 9:00 a.m. - 5:00 p.m. (EST). E-mail address: docdelivery@haworthpress.com].

shelter care between the ages of 7 and 14. At this juncture in their lives, these children are especially open to therapeutic interventions. The authors believe the presented model has application to all racial and ethnic groups, and aspects of the model are applicable to other settings in the foster care system. *[Article copies available for a fee from The Haworth Document Delivery Service: 1-800-HAWORTH. E-mail address: <docdelivery@haworthpress. com> Website: <http://www.HaworthPress.com>* © *2002 by The Haworth Press, Inc. All rights reserved.]*

KEYWORDS. African American male children, foster care, Africentric, model program, disability

Most children enter foster care for reasons of abuse and neglect. Statistics from the Adoption and Foster Care Analysis and Reporting System (AFCARS) indicate there were 568,000 children in foster care for federal fiscal year 1999. This period represents a reported increase of 185,000 from a decade previously. Of the 568,000, 52% were males and 48% were females (National Clearinghouse on Child Abuse and Neglect Information, 2001).

There is concern regarding the increasing number of children of color entering this system and the decreasing number of these children that are exiting. Kellam (2001) cites a report by the W.K. Kellog Foundation published in 2000, which indicates that 57% of children in care are children of color, which constitutes almost twice their representation in the national population (p. 1-2). Of the 568,000 children in foster care on September 30, 1999, 42% were Black (National Clearinghouse on Child Abuse and Neglect Information, 2001).

The Americans with Disabilities Act of 1990 defines disability as: (a) a physical or mental impairment that substantially limits one or more of the major life activities of such individuals, etc. (Pub. L. 101-336). The authors maintain that given the escalating disproportion of children of color in the foster care system, African American children are more prone to being "disabled" in their capacity to be productive and contributive members of society (Morton, 1999).

Brissett-Chapman (1995), via 1994 reporting from the National Clearinghouse on Child Abuse and Neglect Information indicates that:

a. substance abuse and child abuse are strongly linked,
b. these children frequently experienced decreased intellectual functioning, increased disabilities, depression and drug use,
c. long-term pervasive effects of abuse impede mental, physical and social development, which can result in suicide, violence and delinquency,
d. poor people of color are disproportionately subjected to interventions from child protective service agencies (p. 360).

RESIDENTIAL PLACEMENT AND CHILD MALTREATMENT

The history of residential facilities as a means to house and address the needs of children has been controversial. Whether this service is more hindrance than help has been part of the ongoing historical debate. As Whittaker (1995) comments, "[r]esidential provision of any kind today is viewed with extreme suspicion and antipathy. It is often seen as part of the problem and not part of the solution" (p. 449).

Acknowledging the public and professional sentiments toward residential care for children, the authors propose in this article "A Model Program" of care. This model is developed to take advantage of the 24-hour opportunity residential settings provide to positively impact and influence the lives of children. Clearly, residential services are not preferential to children growing up in home environments with nurturing families. However, the authors work from the reality that many children do experience residential care. Consequently, this is a pivotal opportunity for intervention. Based on actual work with African American males, ages 7 to 14, in shelter settings, the authors contend that miracles still do happen and children truly are "a gift of the Creator" when appropriately structured programs are implemented.

Background of Children

Many children who enter residential care, come from economic and emotionally deprived environments. Their neighborhoods reflect racial inequality, which results in city service abandonment and high violence (Seydlitz & Jenkins, 1998). The area probably consists of abandoned houses used as shooting galleries, young men gathering on street corners to sell their products to middle-class white consumers and gangs flourishing as a means of protecting younger children from sexual predators, exploitation and criminal initiation (Harvey et al., 1999).

When mother is a substance abuser or alcoholic, the child's prospects of experiencing a similar outcome are increased (Jenson, 1997). Many of these African American males have had few if any positive African American male role models, as the father is often absent. Many fathers are incarcerated and have little contact with the child. This phenomenon can place the child at risk for becoming a non-constructive adult. Sometimes, the child is living with a grandmother because the biological mother has died from AIDS. Grandmother may request that the child be placed in the care of Department of Social Services because she is no longer physically or financially able to care for the child.

Being African American is a triple whammy for these children (Harvey et al., 1999). First, they suffer the racism that still lingers in a society built on the backs of their forefathers and mothers. Second, they traverse through childhood with little appropriate guidance and support. Last, they lack functional knowledge, understanding and appreciation of African American culture and heritage. A common misperception about these children is that they are slow learners, and academic expectations of them are low (Hilliard, 1997). In the authors' experience, these children are frequently difficult to manage and heavily influenced by the street culture.

Emotional Reaction

Many of these children experience serious psychological problems rooted in their developmental years. Conflict is resolved through either withdrawal or acting out. The acting out usually consists of some form of violence. Snyder et al. (1996) report that in 1994 African American juveniles were six times more likely than their same age Caucasian cohorts to be homicide victims. African American males are placed in the position of fearlessness. As these males strive to survive they can become emotionally anesthetized (Harvey, 1999). Wallen's (1993) research demonstrates that children continually exposed to violence experience symptoms of Post-traumatic Stress Disorder (PTSD). These children harbor constant feelings of being attacked, similar to adults who suffer PTSD (Issaacs, 1992). When these feelings are externalized, they are expressed as angry and raging behaviors. When internalized the children experience depression and are at risk for self-destructive behaviors (Dixon & Ajani ya Azibo, 1998).

Brohl (1996) describes what she calls adaptive responses to traumatic experiences. She contends, and the authors agree, that these are defense mechanisms which guard against experiencing the original physical or psychological pain associated with the trauma. The following are the reactions: rage, aggression, depression, ideation and general listlessness, numbing or blunting, panic attacks, avoidance behaviors, distrust, high-risk behaviors (which may frequently mask depression in African American male youths), sexualized behaviors, flashbacks, sleep disturbances, obsessive-compulsive adaptation, somatic complaints and elimination disorders.

Out-of-home placement can exacerbate a child's reactions. Regardless of the home situation, being removed from familiar surroundings is stressful. The child is removed by an unfamiliar person and can only have fantasies about what to expect. In many cases, he does not know what has happened to his loved ones or what will happen to him. Additionally, he is expected to be grateful and adjust to new rules, new peers and a new school all the while wondering about his future. These children react as they know best–by demonstrating behaviors that keep people at a distance either by being passive or aggressive. A low-level form of aggression is to curse and talk about your mother (Goldstein, 2000). These children know what button to press to set you off. Yet, these are the same children who live with siblings who love each other, know their neighborhood and yearn for adult guidance and a safe place to grow up.

A large percentage of the children have a history of poor school attendance, poor academic performance, and in-school behavioral problems. They are at risk for academic failure and dropping out of school that increases their potential for interfacing with the juvenile justice system (Harvey et al., 1999). These children are to be admired, as they are survivors.

The quality and ability of the shelter to address the psycho-social-emotional-educational-cultural needs of the male child of African descent is crucial in the continuum of care and overall health of the child. It is at this juncture that we have the opportunity to turn a potentially devastating disability into a life success.

Shelter Care Atmosphere

The authors, based on their experience, conclude that the philosophy of many shelter care facilities appears to be that of "warehousing" the youth until they can be placed permanently. Typically, shelters have not developed programs to enhance the academic productivity of the child, nor to address the developmental issues of the child. Staff demonstrates difficulty in discriminating between normal developmental behaviors and trauma response behaviors. In these authors' experience, staff views the child's behavior as "bad" and requiring discipline in the form of punishment. The motif seems to be a reaction to the children as if they are evil and have done something wrong. Staff seems to prefer to hold the children responsible for their situation and use punishment as the primary response to these children. The sad part is that the punishment paradigm is so ineffective with these children because their entire existence has been a semi-punishment. Most have been devoid of rewards and any socially approved reinforce on a consistent basis (Harvey et al., 1999). For punishment to work, children must have phenomena of value in their life. Punishment for these children only reinforces their negative worldview and increases their reactionary behavior. In general, these programs can be said to lack cultural competence (Morton, 1999).

AN AFRICENTRIC PHILOSOPHY

It needs to be stated that an Africentric approach is not only applicable to persons of African descent but is an optimal humanistic approach to living (Meyers, 1988). The central theme of this approach is the mutual responsibility that all human beings have to assist each other in maximizing their "Creator given talents." The process by which this optimally occurs is in an extended family/community/oriented atmosphere (Somé, 1993), inclusive of rituals and ceremonies (Somé, 1998). The adult's task is to build strong bonded relationships with the child and between the children (Hilliard, 2001). The adults form a community of care and establish a safe environment in which children can express themselves and test out their potential talents (Karp & Butler, 1996).

Model Program Goals

Program goals should foster the socialization and normal development of children, providing them with the experience of living in a safe family environment (Hilliard, 2001). The aim is to ensure that the child is better prepared to adjust to his permanent placement. Hopefully, the child will demonstrate a developing ability to establish appropriate relationships, negotiate differences, advocate for himself, and develop critical thinking and appropriate social skills.

The Africentric philosophy driving the shelter's clinical practice recognizes the physically and emotionally traumatic histories of most residents. Many children are diagnosed with Post-traumatic Stress Disorder, Attachment Disorder, Major Depression, or Dysthymic Disorder during their psychiatric evaluation. In response, the shelter is structured to provide a nurturing home environment cognizant of the child's specific developmental stage. Erickson (1968) suggests issues of trust, autonomy, initiative, industry and identity must all be successfully negotiated before the age of 18 years. The shelter program prepares children for successful placement by addressing the risk factors and stimulating the child's sense of personal empowerment. Personal empowerment results from the child's struggle to develop a new repertoire of appropriate behaviors and problem-solving skills.

AN OPPORTUNITY TO GATHER STRENGTH AND HOPE

The following constitutes a condensed view of the referenced program. First, the child meets with the director and case manager. This meeting sets the tone for a new experience. Expectations about his success are described. The support system to ensure this outcome is presented. The strong academic focus of the program is explained. During their 60-day residence, all children attend school. Staff encourage success by creating a nurturing yet accountable environment. The program focus is raising the child's level of critical thinking and problem-solving skills. Through journaling, therapy, "parental discussions" and sharing with peers, the child can develop a vision for his future. Children learn how to operationalize this vision by identifying the immediate goals and behaviors necessary to support the outcomes. Visualization techniques are employed to assist him in this process. Children create collages with pictures of their favorite career, car, and house as part of this process. The finished product hangs in their room. Surrounded by goal reminders, the child learns to have hope.

This program assists the children in developing their own innate skills. Through individual, group and milieu therapy, children begin forming new behaviors. Group therapy presents an opportunity to practice these behaviors.

Typically, these children have become expert in getting kicked out of a facility, whether it is home or school. They appear to have few of the coping skills to stay and invest. The authors maintain that this is both cultivated and reinforced when the child is moved frequently due to acting-out behaviors. The program does not actively focus on extinguishing any of the old behaviors. Rather, the focus is on developing a new repertoire of behaviors, which the child learns to access comfortably over the course of his residence, increasing the probability that old behaviors will be replaced by appropriate ones.

Attachment is encouraged through the use of a system of "good touch." Special handshakes and "safely designed hugs" can allow for a healthy connection between child and staff. Soothing and praise are available, especially comments on the child's ability to regain his composure when agitated. The child is asked to scale the time frame and receives reinforcement for his efforts: "This time you were able to get it together within 10 minutes. Last time it took 25 minutes. What an effort!"

Family Connectedness

Family members are contacted to become part the child's support system. Both the program and philosophy are explained to the family, including the point system. The family is encouraged to call the director to elicit updates on their child's progress in the program. Hopefully, family or caregivers can also contribute to the social, educational and medical history of the child. Family therapy is offered to the family or caregivers.

The process of shaping new behaviors is most effective when the child's efforts are rewarded. The shelter program is based on an elaborate system of rewards that reinforce successful behaviors. The child earns points for completing his daily tasks, including: hygiene, chores, school attendance, homework, and appropriate bedtime behavior. The points are recorded on a large overhead dry-erase board that offers the children a visual picture of their progress to date. The more points the child has, the more money he receives for allowance. Additionally, children earn "Behavior Bucks" for daily completion and return of their individual behavior plan (IBP), successful attendance at group therapy, assisting peers, contributing to the positive atmosphere of the house and demonstrating behaviors which support their personal goal. "Behavior Bucks" can be redeemed for toys, games, clothing, CDs and special privileges, which are available in the house store. As the child becomes more comfortable with his accomplishments, he seems to expect more of the same. He is developing new expectations of himself. Through his struggles, he seems to simultaneously earn a more positive self-view.

Psychosocial

The clinical staff complete a psychosocial by 45 days into placement. This document identifies the various risk factors observed by staff, teachers and doctors. The stimulus for negative behaviors is reported and the specific behavior is described along with the intervention to ameliorate the behavior. The psychosocial is a compilation of this child's known history. A psychiatric evaluation is included. This document is shared with the Department of Social Services (DSS) caseworker in a collaborative effort to identify the most successful placement. The psychosocial contributes to the need for continuity of care. At the juncture of his departure from the shelter there is sufficient information available to allow the placing agency to identify an appropriate long-term placement. The shelter offers step-down services, which are strongly recommended. Here, step-down refers to the gradual process of transitioning a child to his permanent placement while still residing in a safe short-term facility. This process assists the child in making a good adjustment. Additionally, it impedes potential feelings of abandonment.

Strong Academic Focus

Shelter staff dedicate themselves to coaching the child's development of successful school behaviors. This requires constant home-school contact with strong advocacy services in place for the child. Shelter policy requires that each child be enrolled in the local public school within three days of placement. An enrollment package is completed by the case manager that includes a total of 17 documents. The enrollment meeting is used to help the child adjust to the school. He is introduced to his teachers and administrators and he becomes familiar with the layout of the school building. He is usually assigned a class buddy to help him for a few days.

For those children whose behaviors appear unstable and unsafe at intake, a determination is made by the treatment team to send a personal staff member with the child. The staff member rides the school bus and lends support in the classroom and cafeteria settings. Most children enjoy the special attention and it seems an excellent time for developing or strengthening new school behaviors. The staff presence is decreased, as the child's need dictates, until the resident is able to maintain on his own. For those few children who seem unable to function without staff presence, an Arrival, Review and Dismissal Meeting is requested where more intense services are formally considered. The director and case manager are trained as parent surrogates for foster children in the public school system, which accelerates the process. It is unlikely that a new intensity of special education services will be implemented during the child's residence. However, it is likely that the increase in services will be implemented in the long-term placement.

Participation in (and after) school activities is encouraged. Children participate in plays, recitals and sports. These privileges come with a homework mandate, from 3:00 p.m. to 5:00 p.m. on weekdays. Tutors are in place to assist the students and staff is required to review homework for completion. Homework points are awarded, which translate into a bonus in allowance. Shelter individual behavior plans (SIBP), which have been developed by clinical staff, are distributed by morning staff and returned to the afternoon staff. SIBPs contribute to the home-school connection, articulating the child's individual behavioral focus. Children view them as concrete indicators of success, which are connected to rewards. When the sheets have negative teacher comments, the child is able to earn points for bringing the sheet home for discussion. Clinical staff attend parent-teacher conferences and other requested meetings. Teachers and administrators in various local public schools are familiar with the shelter staff and support the program. Shelter staff employ problem-solving techniques on the phone, in the classroom and on the school bus. A new repertoire of tools for problem-solving is not only discussed but also modeled. The resident is aware that someone from his home is advocating on his behalf and he begins to own his share of the work. The child begins to demonstrate the very behaviors that allow him to stay and invest.

African American Role Models and Culture

Ninety-eight percent of the children who are admitted are African American children from the inner city. It is important that the program address the needs of this population (Morton, 1999). Many of these children have not had the benefit of positive role models resembling themselves. The director hires African American males whenever possible, especially mentors knowledgeable in child development and behavioral interventions. It is typical for many discharged children to call staff. In fact, many children refer to a staff member as a family member.

Children are also exposed to African American male role models during career night. Each Wednesday night, a guest speaker is invited into the home. The children prepare the house for the guest and one child has the privilege of introducing the guest. There is also a social opportunity where cookies and punch are set out on a tablecloth with flowers. The speaker shares his personal history and the specifics of his career, including perks and disadvantages. A question and answer period follows the presentation. This sharing of knowledge, success and struggle helps the child determine where he fits in the world. Musicians, policemen, firemen, businessmen, athletes, engineers, doctors, computer technicians, teachers, school administrators, professors and lawyers have all talked with the children.

Rituals and Ceremonies

Knowledge of one's culture with the accompanying feelings of pride can contribute to the development of the child's self-esteem. It is helpful when a child's environment is culturally stimulating. At the shelter, pictures of accomplished African Americans are hung on the walls and field trips to African American museums and institutions are provided.

The value of ceremony and celebration, frequently absent from the child's life, cannot be emphasized sufficiently. The program celebrates birthdays with special cakes and gifts. Successful efforts and outstanding performances are celebrated. All of the typical holidays are celebrated, in addition to Kwanza, an African American Holiday. Children who cannot go to their own homes for Christmas and Thanksgiving are invited into the home of a staff member. Children who do go home bring with them presents from the shelter for the other members of their family. Children also have an opportunity to attend religious services each week. Some of the children participate in activities such as the choir. At discharge there is a ceremony, which includes an exit interview, a departure gift and party. The exit interview includes a review of their academic, emotional and behavioral progress.

RESULTS

The program has been functioning for a year and a half. The authors do not have quantitative data, but estimated and qualitative results exist. At discharge most children demonstrate more appropriate interactive behaviors with peers, staff and other authority figures. Most children become relatively successful students: attend school regularly, remain in the assigned classroom, attempt required work (some receive As and Bs). Most improve their ability to negotiate unstructured environments, such as school bus transportation and school cafeterias. The children are more likely to report a life-long goal and career choice. There is a reduction in the need for physical restraints and an increase in social skills.

POLICY RECOMMENDATIONS

There are implications for policy development on federal, state and local levels. Federal policy should mandate that state and local municipalities increase the educational requirements of shelter staff (a minimum of working toward an Associate degree required for hiring) with equivalent wage compensation. State and local policy should encourage the utilization of culturally-specific service delivery models and develop a tool to measure competency in areas of child development, family interaction and cultural competence. At the program level, staff is evaluated on their intervention skills in working with this population. The quality of the program is determined by the ability of the staff to work effectively with the children. A barrier to quality staff is the high rate of turnover (Coffey, 2001). Some states have created programs to improve compensation (Coffey, 2001). It is critical for children in care to experience a program that maximizes, not disables, the potential for success.

REFERENCES

Brissett-Chapman, S. (1995). *Child abuse and neglect: Direct practice.* Washington, DC: National Association of Social Workers Press.

Brohl, K. (1996). *Working with traumatized children: A handbook for healing.* Washington, DC: CWLA Press.

Child Abuse Prevention and Treatment Act of 1974. P.L. 93-247, 88 Stat 4.

Coffey, K. (2001). Making work possible. *Advocacy [A publication of the Annie E. Casey Foundation], 3,* 16-20.

Developmental Disabilities Assistance and Bill of Rights Act of 1990. P.L. 101-496, 104 Stat. 1191.

Dixon, P. & Anjani Azibo, D. (1998). African self-consciousness, misorientation behavior, and self-destructive disorder: African American male crack-cocaine users. *The Journal of Black Psychology, 24(2),* 226-247.

Erikson, E. H. (1968). *Identity: Youth and crisis.* New York: W.W. Norton & Company, Inc.

Goldstein, A. P. (2000). Catch it low to prevent it high: Countering low-level verbal abuse. *Reaching Today's Youth, 4(2),*10-16.

Harvey, A. R., Coleman, A. A., Wilson, R. & Finney, C. (1999). Psycho-social-cultural needs of African American males in the juvenile justice system. *Journal of African American Men, 4(2)*, 3-17.

Hilliard, A. G., III (1997). *SBA: The reawakening of the African mind.* Gainesville, FL: Makare Publishing Company.

Hilliard, A. G., III (2001). To be an African teacher. *Psych Discourse, 32(8)*, 4-7.

Isaacs, M. R. (1992). *Violence: The impact of community violence on African American children and families.* Arlington, VA: National Center for Education in Maternal and Child Health.

Jenson, J. M. (1997). Risk and protective factors for alcohol and other drug use in childhood and Adolescence. In M. W. Fraser (Ed.) *Risk and resilience in childhood: An ecological perspective* (pp. 117-139). Washington, DC: NASW Press.

Karp, C. L. & Butler, T. L. (1996). *Treatment strategies for abused children: From victim to survivor.* Thousand Oaks: Sage Publications.

Kellam, S. (2001). The color of care: Connect for kids. *Children and Foster Care*, 1-2.

Meters, L. J. (1998). *Understanding an Afrocentric world view: Introduction to an optimal psychology.* Dubuque, IA: Beverly Hills: Sage.

Morton, T. D. (1999). The increasing colorization of America's child welfare system: The overrepresentation of African-American children. *Policy and Practice of Public Human Services, 57*, 23-30.

National Clearinghouse on Child Abuse and Neglect Information. (April 2001). Foster Care National Statistics. Washington, DC.

Seydlitz, R. & Jenkins, P. (1998). The influence of families, friends, schools, and community on delinquent behavior. In T. M. Gullotta, G. R. Adams & R. Montemayor (Eds.) *Delinquent violent youth: Theory and interventions* (pp. 53-97). Thousand Oaks: Sage Publications.

Snyder, H., Sickmund, M. & Poe-Yamagata, E. (1996). *Juvenile offenders and victims: 1996 update on violence.* Washington, DC: Office of Juvenile Justice and Delinquency Prevention, Office of Justice programs, U. S. Department of Justice.

Somé, M. P. (1993). *Ritual: Power, healing and community.* Portland, OR: Swan/Raven.

Somé, M. P. (1998). *The healing wisdom of Africa: Finding life purpose through nature, ritual and community.* New York: Tarcher/Putnam.

Wallen, J. (1993). Protecting the mental health of children in dangerous neighborhoods. *Children Today, 22(3)*, 24-33.

Whittaker, J. (1995). *Children: Group care.* Washington, DC: National Association of Social Workers Press.

Missed Opportunities and Unlimited Possibilities: Teaching Disability Content in Schools of Social Work

Ruby M. Gourdine, DSW
Tiffany Sanders, MA, MSS

SUMMARY. The issue of disability is paramount to the delivery of social services to a vulnerable population–a noble cause of the social work profession. Yet social workers are not the purveyors of services to the disabled. As a way of determining the impact of social work in the field of disability, an analyses of courses are made of disability and school social work content. While this comparison of courses may seem perilous it is important to note that a significant portion of the disabled community are serviced in the schools. The purpose of this article is to raise the professional consciousness of social workers to their responsibility to the treatment and policy development for those who have disabilities. It challenges schools of social work to re-think their course offerings or to reorganize course content to include more information on disabilities. *[Article copies available for a fee from The Haworth Document Delivery Service: 1-800-HAWORTH. E-mail address: <docdelivery@haworthpress.com> Website: <http://www.HaworthPress.com> © 2002 by The Haworth Press, Inc. All rights reserved.]*

Ruby M. Gourdine is Associate Professor, Howard University School of Social Work.
Tiffany Sanders is a doctoral student, Howard University School of Social Work.

[Haworth co-indexing entry note]: "Missed Opportunities and Unlimited Possibilities: Teaching Disability Content in Schools of Social Work." Gourdine, Ruby M., and Tiffany Sanders. Co-published simultaneously in *Journal of Health & Social Policy* (The Haworth Press, Inc.) Vol. 16, No. 1/2, 2002, pp. 207-220; and: *Disability and the Black Community* (ed: Sheila D. Miller) The Haworth Press, Inc., 2002, pp. 207-220. Single or multiple copies of this article are available for a fee from The Haworth Document Delivery Service [1-800-HAWORTH, 9:00 a.m. - 5:00 p.m. (EST). E-mail address: docdelivery@haworthpress.com].

KEYWORDS. Course content on disabilities, social work education, developmental disabilities, school social work

INTRODUCTION

The number of persons with developmental disabilities exceeds 3 million with almost one-half of them needing some type of service during their lifetime (Freedman, 1996). There is a lack of understanding about people who have disabilities because of ignorance of etiology and beliefs about contagion. Therefore, persons with disabilities are often misunderstood and face discrimination (Mackleprang & Salsgiver, 1996) because of fear among the general public. Even though the passage of American with Disabilities Act (ADA) was considered sweeping civil rights legislation, social work as a profession has not yet established itself firmly in the area of policy and services with persons with disabilities.

One may ask the social work profession "who advocates for the disabled (Kirlin, 1985)?" This question is still pertinent as it considers that social work as a profession has not assumed the leadership role in work with this critical population (DePoy & Miller; 1996, Kirlin, 1985; Kirlin & Lusk, 1981). Social work scholars have done little in terms of research and publications on the concerns of the disabled. There are few presentations at national conferences on disability and too few students are encouraged to enter into the field (DePoy & Miller, 1996; Kirlin, 1985; Kirlin & Lusk, 1981). Lack of attentiveness to disability content would appear to have a direct impact on the number of students choosing course work or jobs working with persons who have disabilities.

Given social work's history in administering to the disenfranchised, lack of scholarship and leadership concerning persons with disabilities is both puzzling and disappointing. Previous authors argue that social work has failed to resolve its conflict about this area of service because of internal debates (Kirlin, 1981; Quinn, 1995). Differing perspectives on generic social work versus specialization and the profession's focus on community-based services versus private agencies have fueled this debate. Some of these issues have remained unresolved even into the new millennium.

However, Kirlin (1985) views the unresolved issues as missed opportunities for social work in rehabilitative work. She documents timelines of significant legislation, which represents these missed opportunities for social work. A partial listing follows:

1. 1954 Vocational Rehabilitation Act;
2. 1956 amendments to the Social Security Act provided training funds;

3. 1975 Public Law 94-142, the Education of All Handicapped Children's Act, provides for related services; and
4. 1978 Congress passes Public Law 95-602, title VII of the Rehabilitation Act, Comprehensive Services for Independent Living.

Not only has social work struggled with the issues around disability but also around human and civil rights. Social work has not had a pristine reputation on human rights and civil rights. Although social work purports a perspective of human dignity and worth of the individual, it has been slow to embrace these same standards by promoting diversity and inclusiveness among social work staff, schools of social work faculty and rights of all people. The same laws that were passed to make society more inclusive apply to the social work profession as well. This includes minority groups as well as those professionals who are disabled.

This article will examine the issues surrounding the inclusion of disability content in social work curricula by infusion, specific course work or specific courses, survey schools through Internet listings on the Social Work Action Network (SWAN) and analyze data collected on schools that list content in syllabi or course descriptions.

DEFINING DISABILITY AND DEVELOPMENTAL DISABILITY

Understanding the definition of disability is important in determining the impact content can have on social work curricula. The definitions below provide a framework in which to understand the concept and demonstrate the comprehensive nature and scope of disabilities.

> A Disability is defined as (a) physical or mental impairment that substantially limits one or more of the major life activities of such individual; (b) a record of such an impairment; or (c) being regarded as having such an impairment. (Quinn, 1995 p. 56-57)

> Developmental disabilities are severe, chronic conditions that (1) are attributable to mental or physical impairments or both, (2) are manifested before age twenty-two, (3) are likely to continue indefinitely, (4) result in substantive limitations in three or more major life activity areas (self-care, receptive and expressive language, learning, mobility, self-direction, capacity for independent living, and economic self-sufficiency), and (5) require a combination and sequence of special, interdisciplinary, or generic, care treatment, or other services that are of extended or lifelong duration and are individually planned and coordinated. (Developmental Disabilities Assistance and Bill of Rights Act of 1990 (PL101-496). (Freedman, 1996)

DeWeaver (1996) warns us that definitions of developmental disabilities are often confusing because those that are pre-offered are varied in usage and the intent has differed over time. DeWeaver asserts two major considerations for understanding the term developmental disabilities and they are:

> (1) Definitions are non-diagnostic and focus on what the person can do and skill development, and (2) Definitions move away from the traditional organic model and embrace a social systems perspective which social work endorses. (p. 713)

LITERATURE REVIEW

DePoy and Miller (1996) report that very few schools of social work offer developmental disabilities content in their curricula and those who do, primarily do so through field instruction experiences. Due to a lack of a systematic study of the nature of undergraduate and graduate curriculum content for disabilities, DePoy and Miller (1996) conducted a study of the 498 schools listed in the CSWE directory of which 144 returned their surveys (28.9%). Of those returning surveys, 103 were undergraduate and 36 were graduate schools. Of those studied, 21.53% offered specific courses in disabilities, 88.89% offered field experiences, 59.72% offered research opportunities, but only 3.47% offered a specialization in developmental disabilities. DePoy and Miller conclude that there were more opportunities to study disabilities in graduate schools. Content that was most often covered was disability as a minority status and public policy. This focus is in line with the curriculum policies of the Council on Social Work Education. These authors conclude that social work relies on other arenas to teach social workers about disabilities.

Quinn's (1995) research requested catalogues and admission materials from schools of social work. Her request went to 120 schools and 93 of the schools (78%) submitted course catalogs for content analysis. Of these respondents, 11% or 10 schools focused on disability content in Human Behavior and the Social Environment. Eighteen percent of the schools had policy courses that featured disability content. Policy was covered in 10% (4 schools) of the schools. Thirteen schools or 31% added administration and management courses that included content on disability. In a follow-up survey to faculty from 42 schools (37% responded), she found that the faculty present their content in the foundation courses (infusion) which is endorsed by CSWE and the National Association of Social Workers (NASW).

Limitations in Providing Course Work with the Disabled

Schools of Social Work face limitations in expanding their course offerings, including adding specializations, which may cause problems with turfism and philosophical differences. Another concern has to do with the cost of implementation (Kirlin & Lusk, 1981). Yet another issue is that faculty fail to inform students of opportunities available in the developmental disability areas (DeWeaver, 1996).

Kirlin and Lusk (1981) acknowledge there are still untapped opportunities for students to serve people with disabilities, but were encouraged by social work's role in the area of disability work. Kirlin and Lusk (1981) conducted an exploratory study of both U.S. and Canadian schools. They found that in the United States, a specialization in rehabilitation work was favored by 30% of the U.S. respondents. The Canadians tended to favor multidisciplinary teaching and were able to develop a comprehensive system for working with persons with disabilities. Kirlin and Lusk (1981) recommend that the social work curriculum, with regard to rehabilitation work, would be better served if the student and faculty collaborated in individualized educational planning.

Liese, Clevenger and Haney (1999) concur that schools of social work vary in their ability to practice with persons with disabilities. They recommend that university programs partner with schools of social work to offer curriculum for their students. This recommendation may offer more opportunities for all students at the university but may be difficult to implement. Wysocki and Jamero (1981) assert that social workers have played valuable roles in the field of disability, however, they also acknowledge they have relatively little focus on disability in the graduate schools of social work. Interdisciplinary collaboration is not an easy concept to embrace (Smith, 1996).

Social Work's History in Teaching Disability Content

Kirlin and Lusk (1981) document social work's role in this arena by reviewing the seminal work of Horowitz in 1959. Horowitz was commissioned to conduct a study by the Council on Social Work Education. This three-year study was the first to document the role of social work in rehabilitation work. A major concern identified in this study was whether the content for rehabilitation should be infused in the curriculum, thereby being potentially available to all students, or if in fact it needed to be a part of a specialization. Horowitz (1959) concluded that this content was best offered in a generalist curriculum. In 2001, the question still lingers about how this content should be included in a rather prescriptive social work curriculum. However, if one considers the practicum as a part of the classroom experience, social work actually does quite well as many more students get practicum experience in working with persons with developmental disabilities or other types of disabling conditions (DeWeaver, 1996; Wysocki & Jamero, 1981). The method of providing opportunities through field instruction to students does not seem to be demonstrated in the area of developing leadership because little attention and analysis of these experiences are documented in the literature.

The passage of Americans with Disabilities Act (ADA) facilitated studies of social work involvement in the area of disability (Quinn, 1995). ADA was passed to insure inclusion of people with disabilities in jobs and other social arenas. Social work did pay attention as Tomaszewski (1992) spearheaded an effort to develop a social work disabilities curriculum. DeWeaver and Kropf (1992), Horowitz (1959), and Tomaszewski (1992) propose an infusion model of curriculum to supply disability content. As a result of a grant from the National Institute on Disability and Rehabilitation Research (Department of Education) and the collaboration of the National Center for Social Policy and Practice (NCSPP), the National Association of Social Workers (NASW) and the Washington Business Group on Health (WBGH), a Disability Awareness Curriculum was developed for Graduate Schools of Social Work. According to Tomaszewski (1992), the purpose of this curriculum was to:

1. Facilitate integration and infusion about disability issues into graduate student course work;
2. Be used simultaneously with required foundation areas for master's level social work students to understand the integral place of individual differences and commonalties throughout the entire content of social work education;
3. Offer faculty members the opportunity to address disability issues within their area(s) of specialization; and
4. Provide assistance for graduate schools of social work to develop special-topic courses focused specifically on disability issues (Introduction).

A major concern about expanding curriculum opportunities for students is a relatively low enrollment of students. Is this low enrollment due to low student interest, little to choose from regarding relevant course selection, or low faculty interest in the subject matter?

The Council on Social Work Education elevated to commission status " the Task Force on Social Work Education and Persons with Disabilities" and it was formally recognized in 1995 (a relatively late recognition) (Liese et al., 1999). This action may have more potential for development of leadership in the area of disabilities as it raises the visibility and importance of the issue.

Roles for Social Workers in the Disability Arena

As early as 1959, Horowitz identified the enhancement of the social functioning and family support of the person with a disability as a major contribution of social work. Typically, people with developmental disabilities are poverty stricken or/and rely on governmental programs for assistance (Freedman, 1996). Current social movements in the area of disabilities such as deinstitutionalization and inclusion programs are becoming the norm making it necessary for more social support to help persons with disabilities to be more involved in their communities. "Social workers can play a strong and central role for family-centered practice and collaboration (Freedman, 1996, p. 727)."

DeWeaver (1996) identifies numerous roles for social workers in the area of developmental disabilities. Those roles include: evaluating clients, counseling parents of clients, discharge planning, planners, advocates, protection professionals, providers of direct services or case managers, consultants, resources developers. DeWeaver's (1996) work documented the high level of satisfaction among social workers who work with the population of persons with developmental disabilities. This, of course, is yet another benefit of work with the disabled.

Social workers tend to be regarded as the most appropriate service providers for those with disabilities because of their training in the holistic view of clients, knowledge of resources, skills in commandeering the resources, client advocacy, and knowledge of social policy and laws (Kirlin & Lusk, 1981).

Tempio and Allan (1981) cite the following as functions of social workers working with persons with disabilities:

> (1) Help transition the client from one phase to another; (2) Assist families in mastering the crisis of the acute phrase; (3) Ensures the continuity of relationships during periods of high stress; and (4) Facilitates interactions among health professions. (p. 282)

Limitations that Prevented Social Work from Assuming its Natural Role

The generalist/specialist debate may have negatively impacted social work's role in the area of rehabilitation. The generalists' concept is one of broad knowledge providing the basis of knowing for social workers to work in the rehabilitation field. Specialization is the taking of specific courses to give more in-depth knowledge about a particular subject. Social work's involvement in so many fields limits its ability to be all things to all people and programs (Quinn, 1995). The dearth of rehabilitation professionals results in the hiring of non-professionals or paraprofessionals. Even during professional conferences and meetings little attention is given to the area of disability work. At the annual program meeting (CSWE) from 1989 to 1991 only seven of 500 sessions focused on disability (Resser, 1992).

A review of the literature confirms that social work curricula are pregnant with opportunities that have not yet been translated into the inclusion of more disability curriculum content. There have been some valiant efforts to correct the problem yet the area of disability content in the social work curriculum remains illusive to social work students. There is promise in the field instruction as many more opportunities appear in the practicum experiences. Nonetheless, these opportunities have not translated into leadership possibilities for social workers.

THEORETICAL PERSPECTIVES ON DISABILITIES

Theoretical perspectives provide a framework in which to view disabilities. The life span perspective allows one to view a person across the life span. This is particularly important as improved medical procedures in some instances extended the life span of people with certain disabilities. This perspective includes those persons who may develop a disability during the course of their lives. Further, the move to integrate the disabled in mainstream society requires different types of help to the disabled and their families. The life span perspective explains the needs for those who may have developmental disabilities and their disabilities will not be ameliorated during their lifetime (Freedman, 1996). A case in point is the care for infants and young children who are disabled and their differing needs over their life span.

Tempo and Allan (1981) cite ecosystems as a framework to understand work with persons with disabilities. This approach recognizes the primacy of relationships between the person and their environments in order to understand human functioning. The combination of the bio-pyscho-social experiences is what makes the individual complete. These perspectives embrace the basic tenets of social work, which typically include a holistic view of the person.

RESEARCH QUESTIONS

This article seeks to answer six research questions related to social work curricula content. They are as cited below:

1. How is disability content covered in MSW programs?
2. Do courses focus on a combination of information such as skill and/or policy?
3. Does infused content sufficiently prepare students to work with persons with disabilities?
4. Is there a separation of course content on children and youth versus adults?
5. Is advocacy included as a part of course content on disability?
6. Do schools of social work use interdisciplinary models to teach disability content?

METHODOLOGY AND DATA COLLECTION PROCEDURES

An Internet search was conducted on the MSW and PhD Programs in the United States that were in the Social Work Access Network (SWAN). There were 102 schools listed on SWAN which had MSW or PhD programs in the Unites States; of the 83 of the schools had either course descriptions or catalogues listed on the Internet. An additional search was conducted on all CSWE-accredited MSW and BSW programs. Course content and course listings for disabilities and school social work were extracted. Of the 83 schools included in the survey, 12 (16%) had specially listed courses that covered disability content. Several of the schools listed more than one course on disability; that is probably an indication of specialization of course content. However, for the purpose of this study a school is considered specialized if they had a specific course on disabilities. Similarly, 14 schools listed disability course content for school social work. Again, several schools had more than one course mentioned thus indicating a specialization in school social work.

Although similar methods of data collection have been used before (DePoy & Miller, 1996; Kirlin & Lusk, 1981; Quinn, 1995), the method of an Internet search is a new methodology. The basic tenets were the same as content analysis strategies previously used. The previous studies used mailed surveys and made requests for catalogues and course descriptions. This Internet process has obvious limitations because all schools that have course content on disabilities may not put their catalog or course descriptions on SWAN. Also, course descriptions may not necessarily reflect all the content covered in a course and therefore would not have been used in this study. There may be instances where courses should have been included but were excluded because of the way course content is described. Therefore, this analysis is limited in its generalizability. (See Table 1.)

DATA ANALYSIS

Three of the schools listed provided extensive content on the deaf. One of these schools had seven courses listed for working with the deaf population. One can conclude that perhaps this is a specially targeted program. It is not clear from the catalogues why there is a specific focus on the deaf although one of schools is nationally known for their work with the deaf community. While content on the deaf population is extensive in two of the schools, it is not certain what other disability content is covered. Four of the disability courses were focused on children rather than adults. (See Table 2.)

TABLE 1. Disability Course Content

School Code	Type of Program	Number of Courses	Course Description
001	BSW	3	2 Deaf content 1 overview
002	MSW	2	1 children focused 1 overview
003	MSW	1	1 children focused
004	MSW	1	1 overview
005	MSW	1	1 overview
006	MSW	3	3 deaf content
007	MSW	1	1 children focused
008	MSW	1	1 overview
009	MSW	1	1 overview
010	MSW	3	1 overview 1 specialized content 1 policy
011	BSW/MSW	1	1 children focused
012	MSW	7	7 deaf content 1 human behavior 1 policy 1 micro method 1 macro method 3 field instruction

From a review of literature, courses with a health focus were surveyed in previous research to determine if disability content was included. However, for this article a survey of school social work courses was made primarily because of the passage of the Individuals with Disabilities Act, 1997. This legislation assures that special education services are provided by school districts and specifies the inclusion of social work services. It was assumed for this article that if the course mentioned legal or policy mandates, it would include disability content.

Over fifty percent of the schools (8 out of 14) that had school social work courses also included disability content. These courses probably represent infusion of content in the courses. Additionally, the school social work courses tended to focus on laws and policies. Two courses listed under school social work were also cross-listed in the school of education. One school listed specialized field placements with the deaf population. At least one school social work listing included a doctoral level course that covered disability content. Slightly over 16% of the schools surveyed offered school social work courses.

TABLE 2. School Social Work Course Content

School Code	Type of Program	Number of Courses	Course Description
001	MSW	1	No disability content
002	MSW	1	Disability content
003	MSW	1	Disability content
004	MSW	1	No disability content
005	MSW	2	No descriptions
006	MSW	1	Disability content
007	MSW	1	Disability content
008	MSW	1	Disability content
009	MSW/Ph.D.	3	No disability content
010	MSW	1	Disability content
011	MSW	1	Disability content
012	MSW	3	No disability content
013	MSW	2	Disability content
014	MSW	1	No disability content

DISCUSSION

Disability content is offered in three major ways in the social work curriculum. It is either infused in the curriculum or it is considered a specialization, or a combination of the two methods is used. Few schools seem to cover the content as a specialization. Research in the profession has documented that infusion is the preferred method to impart knowledge on disabilities (DeWeaver & Kropf, 1992; Horowitz, 1959; Tomaszewski, 1992). It is difficult to standardize infusion of content. The argument for the infusion of content is that it reaches more students and the generic courses are appropriate venues for transmission of the knowledge. However, an equally compelling argument against infusion is that it probably does not generate enough interest and skill to provide leadership potential for students in the area of disability work. Students do not see faculty researching, teaching and writing about the subject and therefore are not mentored to develop specific interest in the subject (DePoy & Miller, 1996; Kirlin, 1985).

Courses seem to vary in their presentation from skill development to understanding policy. Advocacy as skill was not articulated in the course outlines or course description, although it would seem inconceivable that advocacy would not be a part of education of social work students.

Some school of social work courses separate out children with disabilities from adults. This method seems to acknowledge the differing needs of these populations. There is some support for interdisciplinary work in the area of disability but there is concern that social work relinquishes its leadership potential by doing this, or an alternative view is that they expand resources by collaboration.

Implications for Social Work Practice

Social work is obligated to cover disability content in its course work. The curriculum policy statements from CSWE require it. Yet each school has the latitude to approach the requirement as it sees fit. Typically two methods used are infusion or specialization. Schools that specialize are regarded as providing intense attention to the area of disability. Schools that approach the disability content by using infusion may be regarded as providing the opportunity for larger numbers of students to learn about disabilities. However, if one supports infusion, it is not clear what standards are used to assure a high level of content. Infusion can be a reading assignment, a lecture, or a classroom assignment. A laissez-faire approach to disability content negates the possibility of developing leadership in the disability arena. The generic approach to school- work requires broad based knowledge from the social worker, possibly making the social worker a jack-of-all-trades and master of none. Yet, given the tremendous social problems, social workers need a generalist perspective. However, the debate on social work's involvement of leadership in the disability arena has gone on too long. This has been problematic, as the profession has missed vital opportunities to provide leadership as researchers, advocates, policy-makers and practitioners.

A recommendation for schools to use interdisciplinary models to supplement content on disabilities is a promising practice, but has some inherent problems as well. There seems to be some precedence for at least considering this model (Liese et al., 1999). The most promising action taken recently in developing leadership is appointing the task force on developmental disability to a Commission within the CSWE. This response elevates the issue to greater visibility both within the profession and to the general public.

CONCLUSION

Social work must make itself more visible in the area of disability work and by doing so become a leader in the field. As it stands now, few schools choose to have specializations in the area of disabilities nor do they typically use a combined model for disability course work. Course descriptions and bulletin write-ups need to be more descriptive. Opportunities to determine interest are missed by students when descriptions fail to tell the whole story about course content. Disability is viewed as a special concern just as racism, sexism and the other isms. To combat these isms is an awesome task for social work. It is one that social work should embrace as its raison d'être. Social work educators should increase the visibility of the profession by increasing disability content in publications and presentations at national conferences. Social workers have had a number of opportunities that have gone unfulfilled. In a profession just past 100 years old, social workers must seize the limitless opportunities the field of disabilities offers as leaders, researchers, advocates and practitioners. It is now time to meet the challenge to become leaders in the area of disability during the 21st century.

REFERENCES

DePoy, E. and Miller, M. (1996). Preparation of social workers for serving individuals with developmental disabilities: A brief report. *Mental Retardation, 34* (1) 54-57.

Devlieger, P.J. and Albrecht, G.L. (2000). Your experience is not my experience: The concept of disability on Chicago's near west side. *Journal of Disability Policy Studies, 11* (1). 51-60.

DeWeaver, K.L. (1996). Developmental disabilities: Definitions and policies. In R.L. Edwards (Ed.), *Encyclopedia of Social Work, 19th Ed*, 712-720.

DeWeaver, K.L. and Kropf, N. L. (1992). Persons with mental retardation: A forgotten minority in education. *Journal of Social Work Education, 28, 36-46.*

Freedman, I. (1996). Developmental direct practice. In R.L. Edwards (Ed.), *Encyclopedia of Social Work, 19th Ed*, 721-729.

Horowitz, J.J (1959*). Education for Social Workers in the Rehabilitation of the Handicapped.* New York: Council on Social Work Education.

Kirlin, B.A. and Lusk, M.W. (1981). Educating social workers for practice in rehabilitation services. In J.A. Browne, B. Kirlin, and S. Watt (Eds.), *Rehabilitation Services and the Social Work Role,* 254-272.

Kirlin, B.A. (1981). Unrealized opportunities: Social work education and the public rehabilitation services. In J.A. Browne, B. Kirlin, and S. Watt (Eds.), *Rehabilitation Services and the Social Work Role,* 332-347.

Kirlin, B.A. (1985). Social work education and services for the handicapped: unfulfilled responsibilities–unrealized opportunities. *Journal of Social Work Education, 21* (1).

Liese, H. Clevenger, R., and Haney, B. (1999). Joining university affiliated programs and schools of social work: A Collaborative model for disabilities curriculum development and training. *Journal of Social Work Education, 35* (1) 63-70.

Mackelprang, R. (1999). *Disability: A Diversity Model Approach in Human Services Practice.* Pacific Grove, CA: Brooks/Cole Publishing.

Mackelprang, R. and Salsgiver, R.O. (1996). People with disabilities in social work: Contemporary and historical issues. *Social Work, 41* (1), 7-15.

Quinn, P. (1995). Social work education and disability: Benefiting from the impact of the ADA. *Journal of Teaching in Social Work, 12,* (1). 55-71.

Resser, L.C. (1992). Students with disabilities in practicum: What is reasonable accommodation? *Journal of Social Work, 28* (1), 98-109.

Smith, J.M. (1996). *A Qualitative Analysis of the Howard University School of Social Work and Education Project.* Washington DC: Howard University School of Social Work and Education Collaboration.

Tempio, C. and Allan, B.M. (1981). Ecological view of social work education in rehabilitation: One school's experience. In J.A. Browne, B. Kirlin, and S. Watt (Eds.), *Rehabilitation Services and the Social Work Role,* 281-287.

Tomaszewski, E.P. (1992). *Disability Awareness Curriculum for Graduate Schools of Social Work.* Washington, DC: National Association of Social Workers.

Wysocki, J.A. and Jamero, P. (1981). Preparing rehabilitation social workers: A curriculum project. In J.A. Browne, B. Kirlin, and S. Watt (Eds.), *Rehabilitation Services and the Social Work Role,* 254-272.

Epilogue

With the expectation that people will be living longer due to new technologies, improved health care and the assertiveness of consumers to make lifestyle changes, the likelihood of more people becoming disabled is almost assured. The request from the disabled is that they are accepted and respected as humans and afforded the same rights and dignity guaranteed to all others. Health professionals and advocates work to keep the larger society and significant resource systems apprised as to the needs of the disabled. They offer recommendations for their assistance with this tremendous task. No one expects that with all that is needed in terms of funding, facilities, resources, practitioners and skilled people, that there can be a change overnight, yet planned change efforts are important. The disabled and their families appreciate the passion and activism for the struggle. Their determination for empowerment and quality of life is evident and espoused by those assisting them. The vision and mission are clear and continue to aid in the successful acceptance and adjustment to disability.

I am deeply appreciative of the wonderful authors who are continuing the struggle to fight for the dignity and rights of the disabled and their families. While recognizing the stressors of disability, the authors have identified and handled the additional issue of race and disability in ways that can heighten understanding and awareness of all helpers. To have valid and reliable information is one of the best efforts in trying to secure and maintain the services and resources needed by the disabled. The advent of additional research can only help to improve what is already available and give optimism to the hard-working advocates trying to continue the already existing atmosphere of empowerment and self-help. It is hoped that others will be encouraged and inspired.

[Haworth co-indexing entry note]: "Epilogue." Miller, Sheila D. Co-published simultaneously in *Journal of Health & Social Policy* (The Haworth Press, Inc.) Vol. 16, No. 1/2, 2002, pp. 221-222; and: *Disability and the Black Community* (ed: Sheila D. Miller) The Haworth Press, Inc., 2002, pp. 221-222. Single or multiple copies of this article are available for a fee from The Haworth Document Delivery Service [1-800-HAWORTH, 9:00 a.m. - 5:00 p.m. (EST). E-mail address: docdelivery@haworthpressinc.com].

http://www.haworthpress.com/store/product.asp?sku=J045
10.1300/J045v16n01_18

The Black community is rich with tradition and culture. With the research showing the inadequacies and disproportionate numbers in all aspects of health and disabling situations of Black life, the community is still hopeful and striving to continue its tradition of strength and courage. There are wonderful models and paradigms and perspectives offered in this volume by the scholars, educators and researchers. The future of the Black disabled community is dependent on the ability to get the results and positions of research and practice wisdoms available to people across all arenas.

I am thankful and appreciative of this team of experts for a job well done. I respect and admire their tenacity in such a difficult field. I commend them for their courage and perseverance.

Sheila D. Miller, DSW

Index

Numbers followed by "f" indicate figures; "t" following a page number indicates tabular material.

Academic achievement, of African American adolescent males, parent-adolescent interaction and, 125-137. *See also* Parent-adolescent interaction

ACF. *See* U.S. Department of Health and Human Services, Administration for Children and Families (ACF)

Acquired immunodeficiency syndrome (AIDS), prevention of, help-seeking and risk-taking behavior among black street youth and, 21-32. *See also* Black street youth

ADA. *See* Americans with Disabilities Act (ADA)

Adams, G.R., 129

Adnopoz, J., 117

Adolescent(s)
African American males, academic achievement of, parent-adolescent interaction influence on, 125-137. *See also* Parent-adolescent interaction
black, help-seeking and risk-taking behavior among, implications for HIV/AIDS prevention and social policy, 21-32
black, help-seeking and risk-taking behavior among, implications for HIV/AIDS prevention

and social policy. *See also* Black street youth, help-seeking and risk-taking behavior among
mental health services for an examination of programs, practices, and policies, 139-153. *See also* Mental health services, for adolescents; Mental health services, for children
barriers to, 143-144

Adolescent-parent interaction, influence on academic achievement on African American adolescent males, 125-137. *See also* Parent-adolescent interaction

Adoption and Foster Care Analysis and Reporting System (AFCARS), 88,196

Adult(s), resident services and programs for, in public housing accommodations, 102-103

Adult Medical Day Care, 102-103

Advisory Commission on Intergovernmental Relations, 6

AFCARS. *See* Adoption and Foster Care Analysis and Reporting System (AFCARS)

Disability and the Black Community

_____ in softbound at $18.71 (regularly $24.95) (ISBN: 0-7890-2077-7)
_____ in hardbound at $29.96 (regularly $39.95) (ISBN: 0-7890-2076-9)

COST OF BOOKS _____

Outside USA/ Canada/
Mexico: Add 20% _____

POSTAGE & HANDLING _____
(US: $4.00 for first book & $1.50
for each additional book)
Outside US: $5.00 for first book
& $2.00 for each additional book)

SUBTOTAL _____

in Canada: add 7% GST _____

STATE TAX _____
(NY, OH, & MIN residents please
add appropriate local sales tax

FINAL TOTAL _____
(if paying in Canadian funds, convert
using the current exchange rate,
UNESCO coupons welcome)

❏ **BILL ME LATER:** ($5 service charge will be added)
(Bill-me option is good on US/Canada/
Mexico orders only; not good to jobbers,
wholesalers. or subscription agencies.)

❏ **Signature** _____

❏ **Payment Enclosed: $** _____

❏ **PLEASE CHARGE TO MY CREDIT CARD:**

❏ Visa ❏ MasterCard ❏ AmEx ❏ Discover
❏ Diner's Club ❏ Eurocard ❏ JCB

Account #_____

Exp Date _____

Signature _____
(Prices in US dollars and subject to
change without notice.)

PLEASE PRINT ALL INFORMATION OR ATTACH YOUR BUSINESS CARD
Name
Address
City   State/Province   Zip/Postal Code
Country
Tel   Fax
E-Mail

May we use your e-mail address for confirmations and other types of information? ❏Yes ❏No
We appreciate receiving your e-mail address and fax number. Haworth would like to e-mail or
fax special discount offers to you, as a preferred customer. **We will never share, rent, or
exhange your e-mail address or fax number.** We regard such actions as an invasion of
your privacy.

Order From Your Local Bookstore or Directly From
The Haworth Press, Inc.
10 Alice Street, Binghamton, New York 13904-1580 • USA
Call Our toll-free number (1-800-429-6784) / Outside US/Canada: (607) 722-5857
Fax: 1-800-895-0582 / Outside US/Canada: (607) 771-0012
E-Mail your order to us: Orders@haworthpress.com

Please Photocopy this form for your personal use.
www.HaworthPress.com

BOF03